*A Woman's Guide to*

*Urinary Incontinence*

# A Woman's Guide to Urinary Incontinence

**RENE GENADRY, M.D.**
Associate Professor of Gynecology and Obstetrics

*and*

**JACEK L. MOSTWIN, M.D., D.PHIL.**
Professor of Urology

Johns Hopkins School of Medicine
Baltimore, Maryland

*The Johns Hopkins University Press*
Baltimore

*This book is not intended to substitute for medical care of people with urinary incontinence, and treatment should not be based solely on its contents. The services of a competent professional should be obtained whenever medical, legal, or other specific advice is needed.*

© 2008 The Johns Hopkins University Press
All rights reserved. Published 2008
Printed in the United States of America on acid-free paper
2 4 6 8 9 7 5 3 1

The Johns Hopkins University Press
2715 North Charles Street
Baltimore, Maryland 21218-4363
www.press.jhu.edu

Library of Congress Catologing-in-Publication Data
Genadry, Rene, 1947–
A woman's guide to urinary incontinence /
Rene Genadry and Jacek L. Mostwin.
    p.   cm. — (A Johns Hopkins Press health book)
Includes index.
ISBN-13: 978-0-8018-8732-1 (hardcover : alk. paper)
ISBN-13: 978-0-8018-8733-8 (pbk. : alk. paper)
ISBN-10: 0-8018-8732-1 (hardcover : alk. paper)
ISBN-10: 0-8018-8733-X (pbk. : alk. paper)
1. Urinary incontinence—Popular works. 2. Women—Diseases—
Treatment—Popular works. I. Mostwin, Jacek L. II. Title.
III. Title: Guide to urinary incontinence.
RC921.I5G46 2007
616.6'2—dc22
2007014818

A catalog record for this book is available from the British Library.

*Illustrations by Jacqueline Schaffer.*

*Special discounts are available for bulk purchases of this book. For more information, please contact Special Sales at 410-516-6936 or specialsales@press.jhu.edu.*

# Contents

Preface   vii

❧ 1 ❧

*Introduction: What Is Urinary Incontinence and
What Can Be Done about It?*   1

❧ 2 ❧

*The Urinary System: Understanding How It Works*   7

❧ 3 ❧

*Stress, Urge, and Mixed: Types of Incontinence
and Their Causes*   16

❧ 4 ❧

*Consulting a Doctor: How to Find the Right Physician
and What You Can Expect*   42

❧ 5 ❧

*Medical Tests: Why and How Are They Done?*   56

❧ 6 ❧

*Nonsurgical Treatments: What Options Are Available?*   68

## 7

*Surgical Treatments: What Does Incontinence
Surgery Involve?* 94

## 8

*Selecting Treatment: Which One Is Right for You?* 125

## 9

*Treatment Complications: What to Do
if Something Goes Wrong* 145

## 10

*Summary: Taking Control of Urinary Incontinence* 162

Glossary 165
Resources 173
Index 177

*Contents*

# *Preface*

You are probably reading this book because you experience urinary incontinence and want to learn more about it or because you are a relative or friend of a woman dealing with incontinence. Urinary incontinence — losing control of the bladder — is common in women. At least one in eight women over the age of 40 will have some degree of incontinence. But incontinence can happen at any age, and it happens for many different reasons. Some women with incontinence will have relatively mild symptoms that they consider a nuisance, while others will have debilitating symptoms that pose a serious problem. In all cases, no matter how mild or severe the incontinence, there are several things a woman can do to improve her quality of life.

Urinary incontinence is an embarrassing problem — nobody wants to lose control over such a necessary but private body function. It was also a relatively neglected problem until recently. However, in 1989, the Agency for Health Care Policy and Research (now the Agency for Healthcare Research and Quality) created an initiative called "Healthy People 2000," which identified a series of major public health problems. One of these was urinary incontinence in adults. Thanks to a growing awareness of the physical problems and social repercussions of urinary incontinence, more and more people — including doctors — are taking incontinence seriously. This is good news for women dealing with incontinence: health professionals are available who understand what incontinence is, what causes it, and how to successfully treat and manage it.

Perhaps you have only recently noticed urine leakage when you participate in certain activities. If that's the case, now is an excellent time to become informed about incontinence — before you seek evaluation and treatment. Alternatively, you may have already been evaluated and tried a treatment that did not work or, worse, had a bad or unexpected outcome. It is never too late to gather information about incontinence and to find out what other options are available. No matter what your situation and background up to this point, you likely have questions about what to do next. Our goal with this book is to help you find answers to your questions — either in these pages or by knowing what questions to ask your doctor — and to help you find your individual path to recovery and health.

In writing this book, we have combined our experience to bring you a comprehensive guide to the causes of and possible treatments for incontinence. We offer information and suggestions about many issues concerning women's incontinence. We also encourage you to become an active partner in your health care and to play a meaningful role in the decisions that will affect your well-being. Nonetheless, we don't intend for this book to replace your doctor. It should help you become better informed about your incontinence and your options, but it should not be used to decide on a treatment without consulting a physician.

Chapter 1 provides some general information about urinary incontinence and what can be done about it. In Chapter 2 we discuss the urinary system and its function because in order to understand what is *not* working correctly in your urinary system, you need to know how it is supposed to work. We then describe, in Chapter 3, the several types of incontinence and the many causes of incontinence, since these pieces of information are critical to finding the right treatment. Chapter 4 discusses finding and consulting a doctor and includes details on what the doctor will ask you and what he or she will do to evaluate your situation. Often, a doctor will suggest that you undergo various medical tests to help make an accurate diagnosis of the type of incontinence; we explain these tests and how they are performed in Chapter 5.

When the doctor has made a diagnosis and you feel comfortable that you fully understand the problem, the next step involves finding out about management and treatment. In Chapter 6, we go through the available options that don't involve surgery, including absorbent products, physical devices, muscle exercises, medications, and injectable materials. In Chapter 7, we discuss the several types of surgical procedures and their success rates; we explain how and why these procedures are done. Knowing what treatments are available is one thing, but considering the benefits and risks of each and determining which will best help you achieve your goal is quite another. Therefore, in Chapter 8, we provide some guidance about selecting the right treatment.

Many of the treatments are reversible — if they don't work or if they cause a different problem, they can easily be stopped. Some treatments — principally surgical ones — are not as easily undone, however, so in Chapter 9 we discuss complications and how they can be addressed. The purpose of this chapter is not to alarm you but rather to ensure that you have all the facts, including those about possible complications, before you decide how to proceed. Chapter 9 will also help you decide what to do if you do have a complication. Chapter 10 concludes the book with a summary of the key points that will help you achieve success in taking back control of your urinary system.

At the end of the book is a glossary of terms, so you can refresh your memory as you read various chapters, and a list of resources to help you find support groups, incontinence products, and further information.

Throughout the book, we tell you the stories of women who have experienced incontinence. Some of these stories may be similar to what you have been going through. They should, at the least, give you a good idea of what you can expect at various stages of dealing with incontinence.

We hope this book will provide you with enough practical information to be able to choose a physician with whom you are compatible, understand the different kinds of incontinence, assess the benefits and risks of various treatments, and participate in the process of addressing your incontinence problems.

*A Woman's Guide to*

*Urinary Incontinence*

## ❧ 1 ❧

## *Introduction: What Is Urinary Incontinence and What Can Be Done about It?*

Every day, more than 12 million Americans, the majority of them women, deal with urinary incontinence. Many people refer to incontinence—which is frustrating and embarrassing—as a "quality of life" issue, but we believe it is considerably more than that. Being incontinent means that you have lost voluntary control over a part of your body that used to function correctly. Regardless of its severity, incontinence can in fact be a personal crisis. With the right information and resources, however, the crisis can be overcome. Incontinence can be managed and in many cases can be partially or totally corrected with treatment. By taking advantage of some of the many options available today, you can resume the lifestyle you had before incontinence began.

### What Is Urinary Incontinence?

Urinary incontinence is the unwanted or unexpected loss of urine. The amount of urine varies from a small leakage that can be absorbed by a thin pad to a large volume that requires more elaborate measures. Incontinence happens to both women and men, although it's more common in women, and it becomes more common as people age. Studies in Sweden estimate that 12 percent of women over age 40 require treatment for urinary incontinence. And the reason for half of all nursing home admissions is that the person has become severely incontinent.

A woman with urinary incontinence suffers more than wetness—she suffers a change in control over her body. The significance of experiencing incontinence should not be underestimated; it can be extremely distressful. Some women, and their families and friends, regard incontinence as a sign of aging or, worse, as a sign of personal deterioration that leads to declining independence. There is no reason, though, for women to lose their independence and curtail all the activities they enjoy simply because of incontinence. Yes, they will likely have to make adjustments, and they may decide to go through medical treatment that has physical, emotional, and financial impacts. But support, information, and medical resources are available to help women dealing with incontinence.

People cope differently with incontinence. For some it is a nuisance, but they make adjustments and continue their daily activities; for others it is a disaster that disrupts or ends their social or professional life. Some women successfully manage fairly severe incontinence, but others limit their activities with even a small amount of incontinence. For example, compare the stories of Sally and Lynne.

*Sally, who experiences incontinence that requires frequent pad changes, left her job as a high school art teacher because she was constantly afraid of losing bladder control and didn't trust the pads to absorb the urine or to be invisible under her clothing. She now teaches art classes for adults and children from her home, where she can more easily run to the toilet. However, she makes much less money than in her previous job, and she misses the professional interaction with other teachers.*

*Lynne is a real estate agent in her early fifties and has experienced incontinence for several years. She wears pads and has to change them about every two hours during the day. Even though her work means that she is frequently away from her office, she knows where to find all the public toilets in the city. She keeps spare pads in her car as well as in her purse, and she wears skirts and dresses instead of pants. Lynne has had to make some adjustments, but she continues to enjoy her active professional life.*

Incontinence is not a disease but rather a symptom of an underlying condition, so it happens for a variety of reasons. One of them certainly is age, but age is often incorrectly blamed. There are many other causes of urinary incontinence:

*A Woman's Guide to Urinary Incontinence*

- Urinary tract infections
- Pregnancy and childbirth, which can cause temporary incontinence as well as weakening of the pelvic-floor muscles, increasing the possibility of a woman's developing incontinence later in life
- Menopause
- Conditions such as diabetes, multiple sclerosis, and stroke
- Spinal cord injuries and injuries to the pelvic region
- Pelvic surgery
- Medications for other conditions
- Obesity

The severity of incontinence and the rate at which it progresses, or improves with treatment, depend on several factors, such as age and weight. With age, muscles weaken, and it takes more time to re-strengthen them with exercises. Being overweight can exacerbate stress incontinence, which occurs when a person sneezes or coughs, for example.

## What Can You Do about Incontinence?

Many women who experience bladder problems suffer in silence. They are too embarrassed to mention their incontinence to a doctor, or they think nothing can be done to alleviate the problem. Yet the majority of women with incontinence can expect to have their problem improved, if not eliminated, provided the cause is diagnosed and thoughtfully selected therapy or treatment takes place. At the very least, women who seek help will have a greater understanding of their problem and of the possible options to help them develop better control. To find the path to improving an incontinence problem, a woman needs to approach her health issues actively. She can seek support from family and friends, get help from counselors and medical professionals, become informed about options for management and treatment, define her goals and priorities, and decide how far she wants to go in resolving her situation.

If you experience incontinence, the first step is to realize that you are not alone and that help is available. If you can, talk to one or a few family members or close friends so that they know what you are going through. For many women, telling others about their problem eases the embarrassment they feel. Ask the person you confide in for help and support, whether it be giving advice, helping you find out your options, or simply listening to you. Don't underestimate the healing power of telling your story to a sympathetic person. You may also ask a family member or friend to drive you to appointments with your doctor or to take care of daily chores while you attend appointments, undergo treatment, or recover from an operation. Asking someone to handle appointment bookings and medical bills while you concentrate on recovery may also be of great help.

Some people prefer to face their problems alone or don't want to involve their family or friends. In these situations, there are other people you can turn to for help, including specialized counselors, social workers, and chaplains or pastoral counselors. Attending a support group can be a great way to share your story and get information from others experiencing the same or similar problems. Contact some of the organizations listed in the Resources at the back of this book to find a counselor or support group in your community. If you find that your reaction to incontinence dominates every other aspect of your life, then psychiatric counseling, and sometimes medication, may help you cope. Your primary-care physician should be willing to discuss your situation and refer you to a psychiatrist if you need this kind of help.

No matter whom you choose to turn to or confide in, go to a doctor to explain the problems you're having and begin finding answers to your questions. The right doctor can evaluate you, make a diagnosis, and describe the many options for managing and treating incontinence. These options include lifestyle changes, exercises to strengthen the pelvic-floor muscles, medication, surgery, and others, some of which require minimal intervention and have few or no side effects. Some options can be provided by a family doctor, while others require the expertise of one or more specialists.

As well as consulting a doctor about your incontinence, we encourage you to learn as much as possible about the problem and what can be done about it. Being well informed makes you a partner in your health care, improves your ability to understand and communicate with your doctor, and promotes realistic expectations of treatments. As doctors who help women with incontinence every day, we are always encouraged by a woman who seeks information to understand the implications of her symptoms both for the present and for the future.

Armed with information, you will be in a good position to make decisions about your situation and about how to proceed in your efforts to overcome the problem. The doctor's role is to make a diagnosis and to discuss your options with you; he or she can make recommendations but cannot decide what action will work best for you. Unfortunately, some people make inappropriate decisions because they don't have enough information or because they don't consider all the available information from the perspective of their situation. It can be easy to be swayed by the experiences of friends and family or by advertisements for the latest product or treatment, but keep in mind that incontinence happens for many reasons, so what works best for you may differ greatly from what works for other women.

To make the best decisions about your health care, you also need to be fully aware of your priorities. For example, one woman may decide that it's more important for her to attend to a child's or other family member's needs than to undergo an operation. Another woman may prefer to gain partial improvement through a lower-risk option than to possibly achieve a permanent cure through a higher-risk option.

When trying to resolve an issue like incontinence that can so severely affect your quality of life, it is essential to set goals for your recovery. Depending on the cause of your incontinence and the treatment you select, you may return to the kind of urinary control you had before the incontinence began. However, this outcome is not realistic in every situation, and so you may experience only a partial return to your previous state of health. If you can determine what you want to achieve and what is realistic in your situation before embarking on a treatment plan, then you are most likely to be successful in reaching your goals. Before you make a decision to undergo any particular treatment, write down your view of success from that treatment and discuss it with your doctor. Be sure that you and the doctor agree that the result you seek is possible given the cause of your incontinence and the treatment option you have selected. Also think about how much time you are willing to spend trying various treatments in case the first one doesn't work as well as expected. You may find that you will have to adjust some of your recovery goals or explore other management or treatment options to achieve success and maintain a quality of life that you want.

Regardless of how large or small your problem with incontinence is at the moment, you can take charge of your situation by finding out as much as you possibly can and by seeking medical evaluation. Don't restrict your activities and put up with incontinence because you think there are no other options; there are many options, and they are waiting for you to explore them.

## ❧ 2 ❧

# *The Urinary System: Understanding How It Works*

T he urinary system includes two kidneys, two ureters, the bladder, and the urethra (Figure 1). The kidneys make urine, which the tubelike ureters transport into the hollow bladder for storage. When the bladder is emptied, the urine flows through the urethra, a short muscular passage that connects the bladder to the outside of the body. The muscles surrounding the urethra, called the urethral sphincter muscles, constrict to help keep urine in the bladder while it fills and relax when the bladder contracts and expels urine. Another set of muscles, the pelvic-floor muscles, supports the bladder and the urethra within the pelvis. The pelvic-floor muscles can be thought of as a hammock attached to the bones in the pelvis. The bladder and urethra, as well as the vagina and rectum, are suspended in the hammock. In this chapter, we describe in more detail how the organs and muscles of the urinary system function and coordinate to make, store, and release urine.

## The Kidneys: Where Urine Is Made

The kidneys are bean-shaped organs, each one about the size of your open hand. They are located in the back of the abdomen, behind the digestive organs, a few inches inside the space protected by the lowest two or three ribs. The kidneys filter waste products out of the blood 24 hours a day. This is done by means of hundreds of square feet of a wafer-thin tissue, much like cheesecloth, crinkled up into tiny spaces inside each kidney. When the blood passes across this

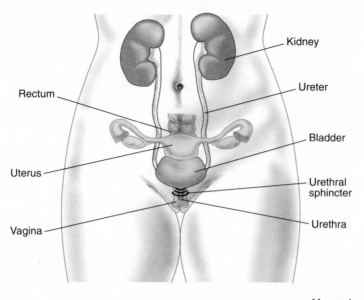

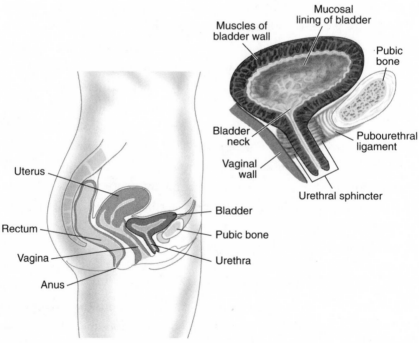

Figure 1. The urinary tract: the kidneys, ureters, bladder, and urethra

tissue, excess water — along with dissolved waste products that the body must dispose of to remain healthy — is removed from the blood. This mix of water and dissolved waste products undergoes some additional processing before it leaves the kidneys as urine. The urine travels down one of two thin, muscular tubes called the ureters, each one 23–30 centimeters (about 9–12 inches) long, on its way to the urinary bladder. When a person ingests a normal amount of fluid — about 2,000 milliliters (½ gallon) per day — the kidneys will typically produce 800–1,600 milliliters (⅕ to ½ gallon) of urine during the day.

## The Bladder: Where Urine Is Stored

The bladder, which is shaped like an inverted balloon, can usually accommodate a significant volume — between 300 and 600 milliliters (between 10 and 20 ounces). The neck of the bladder tapers, ending in a short snout called the urethra. In adult women, the urethra is about 4–5 centimeters (1½–2 inches) long. The urethra and the tapered part of the bladder are firmly fixed in position by ligaments (fibrous bands of tissue) between the pubic bone and the front wall of the vagina. The rest of the bladder is arranged in such a way that it can stretch up into the abdomen as it fills with urine.

The walls of the bladder are made up mostly of muscles, but they are not like the muscles in your arms and legs. You cannot make the bladder muscles contract or relax at will. They are one of the many involuntary muscles that are under automatic control by the body. Other involuntary muscles in the body include the muscles of the digestive tract, the muscles surrounding arteries and veins, and the muscles of the uterus. Because of the way these involuntary muscles look under a microscope, they are called smooth muscles. This description distinguishes them from the voluntary muscles of the body, which have thin black bands when viewed under a microscope. Because of these bands, voluntary muscles are called striated (striped) muscles.

Smooth muscles are capable of stretching farther and contracting longer than striated muscles. If the muscle of your forearm were stretched only 20 percent as much as a strip of bladder muscle, it would be ripped apart. Striated muscles are generally more powerful and are quicker to contract and relax than smooth muscles, and as already mentioned, striated muscles are under voluntary control. That's why you can hold this book in your hand and turn this page.

As the bladder fills with urine, the smooth muscles stretch to accommodate the urine, and the bladder enlarges. Because of the elastic capabilities of the smooth muscles, the bladder's internal pressure during the filling phase normally stays low. However, when the bladder muscles contract to expel urine, the pressure inside the bladder rises. Once the bladder is emptied, the smooth muscles return to their unstretched state, and the bladder pressure subsides.

## The Urethra and Urethral Sphincter

Like the bladder, the urethra is made up of smooth, involuntary muscles. The muscles of the urethra are a continuation of the bladder muscles. The arrangement of the muscle fibers results in a narrow, tapered shape where the bladder funnels into the urethra, sometimes also called the bladder neck (see Figure 1). The urethra remains tightly closed when its smooth muscles are at rest, or relaxed. (The urethra opens when the bladder muscles contract and pull the urethral walls away from the center of the tube.) The tube of the urethra also has smooth muscles along its length to help to keep the urethra closed. Along with the muscles, blood vessels in the urethra contribute to the seal that blocks urine from leaking out. Estrogen helps to maintain these blood vessels and the muscles in the urethra, so the lack of estrogen after menopause can lead to increasing problems with incontinence. Surgery, radiation therapy, and vaginal delivery can also damage the urethra and reduce its ability to stay tightly closed.

The urethra is surrounded by a sleeve of striated muscles called the urethral sphincter (Figure 2). Unlike the smooth muscles of the bladder and urethra, the urethral sphincter is under voluntary control. The urethral sphincter remains closed to keep urine in the bladder when there is physical stress within the abdomen (such as when you sneeze or lift a heavy object) or when some urine has leaked into the upper portion of the urethra. The sphincter basically pulls upward and forward on the urethra and "milks" the urine back into the bladder. Childbirth, pelvic surgery, aging, and menopause can all affect the ability of the urethral sphincter to constrict the urethra.

*A Woman's Guide to Urinary Incontinence*

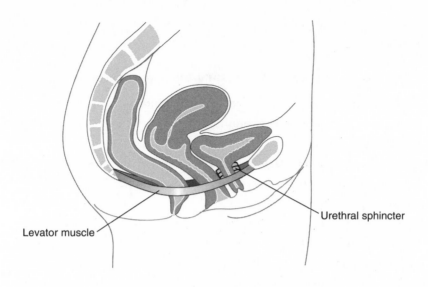

Levator muscle

Urethral sphincter

Figure 2. The urethra and its sphincters

## Pelvic-Floor Muscles

The pelvic-floor muscles, also called the levator muscles from the Latin word for lifting, line the inside of a woman's pelvis and provide support to the urethral tube and to the bladder, vagina, and rectum. Each of these pelvic organs opens to the outside of the body, through a gap in the pelvic floor. The pelvic-floor muscles, which are striated and therefore voluntary muscles, form a bowl lined with parallel slings that attach to the pelvic bones and to the edges of the connective tissue (see Figure 2). When these muscles contract, they pull from back to front, lifting the pelvic organs forward and closer to the pubic bone. Because of their position and the fact that they are striated muscles, the pelvic-floor muscles are vulnerable to overstretching during pregnancy and childbirth. When the pelvic muscles have been stretched, they provide less support for the urethra so that urine can leak more easily through the urethral tube. Also, with less support from the pelvic muscles, the bladder and other pelvic organs can slide out of their normal position and move closer to the vaginal opening, a condition called prolapse. Kegel exercises, which are familiar to many women who are trying to overcome incontinence, involve the voluntary contraction and shortening of these pelvic-floor muscles to strengthen and reeducate them.

## The Cooperation of Voluntary and Involuntary Muscles

For the most part, the organization of voluntary muscles is separate from the organization of involuntary muscles. Conscious parts of the brain regulate voluntary muscles, while unconscious parts of the brain regulate involuntary muscles. In a few situations, though, voluntary and involuntary muscles must work together to achieve a common goal. Swallowing is one of these situations: the voluntary swallowing muscles of the throat and upper esophagus (the swallowing tube) must work in harmony with the involuntary muscles of the lower esophagus to deliver food to the stomach. Urination is another: the voluntary muscles of the urethral sphincter and pelvic floor must work together with the involuntary muscles of the urethra and the bladder to release urine when the person wants to release it.

Muscle function is controlled by nerves — delicate cables that convey information to and from the brain. Smooth, involuntary muscles and striated, voluntary muscles are controlled by different parts of the nervous system and are supplied by distinctly different nerves (Figure 3). The voluntary muscles of the urethral sphincter and the pelvic floor are linked to the central nervous system by the two pudendal nerves, one on each side of the body. These nerves enter the pelvis through small openings in the bone at the back of the pelvis and travel underneath the pelvic floor to connect with the muscle fibers of the urethral sphincter and the pelvic floor. Each pudendal nerve is stretched like a tightrope from the back of the pelvis to the front. Its position makes it vulnerable to damage during childbirth.

A completely different nerve supply connects to the smooth muscles of the bladder and urethra. These muscles are supplied by the two pelvic nerves, again one on each side of the body. Each pelvic nerve travels right along the central edge of the pelvic opening, giving off smaller branches to the rectum, uterus, bladder, and urethra. Because the pelvic nerves are close to the pelvic organs, they can be easily injured during pelvic surgery or radiation therapy.

The control center coordinating nerve signals and the interaction

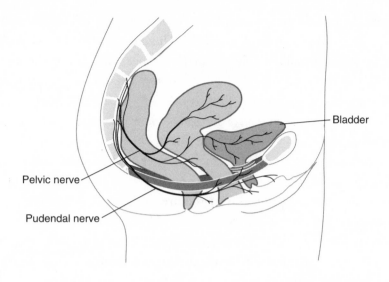

Figure 3. The nerves to the bladder, urethra, and urethral sphincter

of voluntary and involuntary muscles is located at the base of the brain, in the brain stem. It is a long way from the control center in the brain to the lowest reaches of the pelvis; signals have to travel up and down the entire length of the spinal cord. Along the way, there are a number of relay stations where information is shared between the nerves supplying the voluntary muscles and those supplying the involuntary muscles.

## The Bladder Cycle

The bladder cycle refers to urine filling the bladder, being stored in the bladder, and being emptied from the bladder. The bladder spends 99 percent of its time resting and slowly stretching as urine trickles into it. The urethra normally remains closed throughout this entire time. The bladder can accommodate a substantial volume of urine — up to 600 milliliters (20 ounces) under normal conditions — before the feeling of bladder fullness peaks. It doesn't seem as though much is happening during this filling phase, but in fact a lot is going on. As the bladder stretches, it sends a slowly increasing signal to the control center in the brain stem. The brain stem passes the signal to the conscious part of the brain, and the brain responds by slowly increasing the tension in the urethral sphincter. The more the bladder stretches, the stronger the signal going to the brain becomes, and the more the tension of the urethral sphincter increases. The increasing tension of the sphincter is also transmitted from the brain stem through various relay stations in the spinal cord to the bladder nerves to block the competing signals that are encouraging the bladder to contract and empty.

Eventually, the signals become strong enough that the person feels an urge to urinate. A person with normal urinary function will find a toilet and maintain control over the urethral sphincter until it is time to relax it and urinate. By consciously relaxing, the person voluntarily allows the pelvic-floor and sphincter muscles to go limp. As these muscles relax, the bladder neck rotates downward, the urethra descends in the pelvis, and the urethral tube opens (Figure 4). At this point, the bladder muscles begin to contract and shorten, funneling urine out through the open urethra. The urethra transmits information about the continuous flow of urine back to the brain, ensuring that the bladder muscles keep contracting until all the urine has been expelled. Once the bladder is empty, the bladder muscles relax, the urethra returns to its closed resting position, and the bladder starts to fill again for the cycle to repeat. As long as the kidneys produce urine, the bladder cycle will continue.

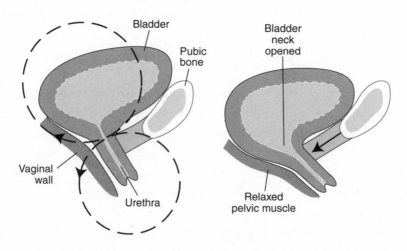

Figure 4. Rotational urethral descent during normal voiding

*A Woman's Guide to Urinary Incontinence*

## Toilet Training and Bladder Control

Most people learn to recognize the subtle signals that come from the bladder as it fills and learn to activate and maintain tension in the urethral sphincter muscle between the ages of 2 and 4, the common time of toilet training. Before then, the nerves required to deliver the signals to and from the sphincter muscles have not matured enough to function properly. In babies and young children who aren't yet toilet trained, the bladder fills to a certain volume and then empties by a reflex that can sometimes be provoked by touching or stroking the lower abdomen or genitalia. Anyone who has changed the diaper of a baby boy is familiar with this reflex. The reflex cannot be voluntarily suppressed.

Only when the nerves controlling the voluntary muscles have matured can toilet training be learned. For elderly adults who have lost awareness of bladder sensation and the events of the bladder cycle, repeating the lessons of toilet training learned in childhood is a way of helping to regain some control. The ability of an adult to relearn this kind of control depends on the health of the nerves carrying the signals, the strength of the sphincter muscles and reflexes, and the alertness of the brain.

When it is impractical or impossible to find a toilet, the normal reaction is to try to tighten the muscles of the pelvic floor in an attempt to hold back the urge. This is successful in the early stages of bladder filling. At later stages, it becomes more difficult. With training, this effort to tighten the muscles can be made into an effective method for dealing with urgency and even urge incontinence.

This brief overview of the urinary system and how it functions should give you enough information to understand what happens when the urinary system doesn't function correctly, which is the subject of the next chapter.

## ❦ 3 ❦

# Stress, Urge, and Mixed:
# Types of Incontinence and Their Causes

For the urinary system to function correctly, a variety of muscles and nerves must do their jobs in a coordinated way, as described in Chapter 2. If a single element in the system is not functioning as it should, the result can be incontinence. There are two common types of incontinence: stress incontinence, which happens when an activity or event increases the pressure in the abdomen and the bladder can't resist the extra pressure; and urge incontinence, which happens when a woman has a strong desire to urinate and she is unable to stop urine from leaking out. Some women experience mixed incontinence, which means they have symptoms of both stress and urge incontinence, with one usually being dominant. Another, less frequent type is overflow incontinence, in which the bladder doesn't empty completely and urine spills out as the bladder refills. Finally, there are a few other infrequent types of incontinence that result from abnormalities of the urinary system. For example, the urethra sometimes has a small pouch or pocket in it, called a diverticulum; the bladder and vagina are sometimes connected by a tunnel or passage that shouldn't be there, called a fistula; and sometimes a girl is born with a urethra that has failed to close, a condition called epispadias.

We begin this chapter with a description of each type of incontinence, including the symptoms and general causes. Then we discuss various conditions and factors that can lead to incontinence.

## Stress Incontinence

The most common form of incontinence in women is stress incontinence, which occurs with physical stress. In this case, the bladder often functions entirely normally until it is subjected to a stressful event that increases pressure in the abdominal cavity. Familiar activities that bring about increases in abdominal pressure are coughing, sneezing, laughing, jumping, jogging, and having sexual intercourse. Any of these activities may overcome the urethra's ability to remain closed and retain urine in the bladder (Figure 5). Stress incontinence occurs when urethral resistance to leakage decreases as urinary bladder pressure increases in response to abdominal pressure. Changes in urethral resistance during stress are caused by the combined effect of weakened vaginal support (prolapse) and weakness of internal urethral structures (so-called ISD — intrinsic sphincter deficiency). Determining how much of the leakage is due to urethral weakness and how much is due to vaginal weakness is a critical part of medical testing described in Chapter 5, "Medical Tests: Why and How Are They Done?"

An increase in abdominal pressure squeezes the bladder and the urine it contains, as well as the other pelvic organs and muscles. If the walls of the urethra and the tissues supporting the urethra are weak, the pressure transmitted to the urine in the bladder will simply push apart the walls of the urethra. Most frequently, the urethra is unable to stay closed because it is not well supported by the surrounding pelvic-floor muscles and connective tissue, and so the urethra becomes more mobile than it should and opens more easily. A sudden increase in abdominal pressure is enough to push the urethra and bladder out of their normal location and put enormous strain on the urethra's regular ability to remain closed. The second line of defense — the urethral sphincter — can sometimes contract enough to counteract the urethra's mobility and inopportune opening. If the sphincter can't constrict tightly enough, though, incontinence occurs.

It is usually not possible to tell that the urethra has lost support and become more mobile — in other words, you won't feel it moving.

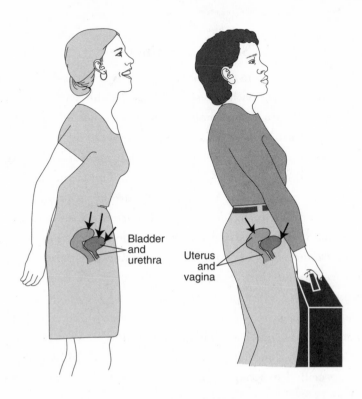

Figure 5. Direction of force on bladder from activities that
provoke stress incontinence

In severe cases, a slight bulge may be felt at the entrance of the
vagina, just inside the vaginal opening. The bulge becomes more no-
ticeable when a woman strains or coughs because the increased pressure in the abdomen pushes the bulge beyond the vaginal opening.
As described in Chapter 4, a physician uses a cotton swab inserted in
the urethra as one way to determine whether the urethra is mobile.

Stress incontinence may begin during or shortly after childbirth or
shortly after menopause. In the beginning, it may occur only with
strenuous exercise and later with laughing, coughing, or sneezing. As
it becomes worse, it can occur with a movement as simple as standing
up from a chair with a full bladder, bending over to adjust a shoelace,
picking up a child, or even turning over in bed.

For many years, it was thought that childbirth was the primary
factor causing the development of stress incontinence. More recent

*A Woman's Guide to Urinary Incontinence*

studies suggest that it's not so simple. Pregnancy itself may be a factor because of the enlarged uterus and the hormonal changes that affect all tissues of the body at this time. Several other factors, particularly those that raise the pressure in the abdominal cavity, favor the development of stress incontinence. These include frequent coughing from chronic bronchitis, asthma, or other lung problems. Smoking, of course, contributes significantly to these problems. Constipation and the need to strain during bowel movements can weaken support within the pelvis by stretching both muscles and nerves. Estrogen deficiency, which can occur during menopause, affects the elasticity of the connective tissues, as do trauma, surgery, and radiation therapy. Aging brings about a decline in the mass and strength of muscles and connective tissue, and many years of gravity pulling on internal organs and other structures may play a role in developing stress incontinence. Some women also may have inherited a connective tissue weakness. Finally, environmental factors, particularly jobs that require a lot of straining or lifting, can contribute to the development of stress incontinence. In any one person, several of these factors may each contribute a small part toward developing incontinence, and together they add up to a large effect on the ability of the body to retain continence.

## Urge Incontinence

As the name implies, urge incontinence is associated with a powerful and often unexpected need to urinate. The symptom of urgency is not simply an exaggerated version of the normal feeling a woman has when her bladder is full but rather an overwhelming sense of needing to urinate immediately. Urge incontinence typically also involves a sudden loss of urinary control. Many women report that they suddenly develop a strong urge to empty their bladder and they start to leak or even lose complete control before they are able to get to the toilet. Some women find they are powerless to stop urination if they put their hands into water or even if they hear the sound of running water. Others feel a sudden, strong urge as they return home and put the key in the door; unable to control the urge, they struggle to run to the toilet or stand powerless as urine leaks out. Sometimes, a woman will experience the urge to urinate only seconds before realizing that she has wet herself. Urge incontinence happens most often during the day, but some women wake up at night with a strong need to urinate, a symptom called nocturia. The term *enuresis* is used to describe the condition when a person wets the bed at night — the same term applies to both adults and children.

Urge incontinence is the involuntary loss of urine associated with an irresistible desire to urinate. At times, the slow buildup of signals doesn't happen, so the woman doesn't get advance warning of needing to empty her bladder. Instead, a sudden signal from the nervous system causes the bladder's smooth muscles to contract. The contraction may overcome the urethral sphincter or lead to normal relaxation of the urethra to expel urine.

Urge incontinence can have many different causes, and it can be hard to pin down exactly why it's happening. Urge incontinence commonly occurs when a woman has a bladder infection (cystitis), urinary tract infection, or bladder stones; occasionally it occurs with bladder cancer. It is also a common symptom in people with an illness or injury affecting the neurological system (such as Parkinson disease), the brain (such as a stroke), or the spinal cord (such as multiple sclerosis).

Until recently, urge incontinence was attributed primarily to an irritation of the bladder or to a change in the nerve control of the bladder, both of which increase the bladder's sensitivity. However, it now appears that urge incontinence may often be related to stress incontinence. In this case, the symptoms of urgency coexist with stress incontinence, and both types of incontinence result from weakness of the urethra. In many women with this mixed incontinence, the urine forced into the urethra by increased abdominal pressure triggers a reflex for the bladder to contract. Normally, the reflex would be suppressed by voluntary contraction of the urethral sphincter, but if the sphincter is weak or impaired, then the bladder will start to empty and cannot be stopped. The increased pressure causes the stress incontinence, and the sudden bladder contraction causes the urge incontinence. Frequently, targeting the stress incontinence by strengthening the urethra also stops the urgency symptoms.

## Overflow Incontinence

Overflow incontinence means exactly what it says: the bladder over-flows and urine leaks out. It usually occurs when the bladder does not empty completely — because of weak bladder muscles or impaired urination reflexes — so that as the bladder refills, it quickly reaches its capacity and excess urine overflows. Some people with overflow in-continence will feel the urge to urinate, but the urge occurs later than normal or when leakage has already started. Because the bladder fills to capacity, there is also some danger of urine being forced back up the ureters toward the kidneys, but this is exceptionally rare in adult women. Overflow incontinence may result from several circumstances, including when a woman has sustained injuries in the pelvic region, when she has congenital anomalies of the lower spine, or when she has a weak urethra with poor bladder sensation.

## The Overactive Bladder

You may have heard the term *overactive bladder* and wonder how it fits into the types of incontinence described here. *Stress, urge,* and *overflow incontinence* are terms that arose in the medical profession in an era when physicians studied and classified illnesses. The term *overactive bladder,* however, arose more recently, when newer drugs were be-coming available for the treatment of urinary tract symptoms. The term was coined to simplify the description of the condition to be treated and to avoid direct links to the older medical terms. Using the term made it easier for treating physicians to create a category of people who could be offered a single drug for treatment.

*Overactive bladder* is the term used to describe the condition experi-enced by people with frequent or urgent urination, whether or not they experience incontinence. A woman described as having an over-active bladder may or may not be incontinent. If she is incontinent, she will experience urge incontinence. If she isn't, she will experience symptoms of urgency and will feel the need to urinate frequently. Some women with an overactive bladder, with or without urge incon-tinence, may also experience stress incontinence.

It can be difficult to tell whether a woman's urgency is caused by a contracting bladder or by urine passing through a weakened urethra. This difficulty lies in the fact that the bladder and the lower urinary tract are primitive structures within the overall nervous system. There are only so many nerve fibers and impulses that can travel back and forth from the brain and the higher control centers to the bladder, urethra, and pelvic muscles. Therefore, many different kinds of events in the pelvis can give rise to the same feeling of urgency. A bladder that is too sensitive and wants to empty suddenly before it has filled will produce the same kind of urgency symptom as a bladder that has lost its sensation and experiences urgency only when the accumulated urine starts to spill over into a weakened urethra. Either way, the person experiences the sudden need to run to the toilet, or she feels urine coming and can't stop it. Unfortunately, urgency is one of the most frustrating symptoms to experience because it is poorly understood and therefore can be difficult to treat.

## Incontinence with Bladder Infections

Any source of irritation in the bladder — including bladder infection, stones, or cancer — can cause symptoms of frequency, urgency, or both. An irritated bladder may cause the smooth bladder muscles to contract strongly and overwhelm the normal continence mechanisms. The result is incontinence, usually urge incontinence. The incontinence can generally be resolved, however, by removing the irritant from the bladder. In the case of a bladder infection, the treatment involves antibiotics, which usually cure both the symptoms and the incontinence itself.

## The Effects of Pregnancy and Childbirth on Incontinence

Any woman who has been pregnant knows that pregnancy often means more frequent trips to the toilet. As the uterus enlarges with the developing baby, it presses on the bladder and causes the sensation of needing to urinate (Figure 6). The bladder becomes more sensitive and its capacity decreases, leading to the frequent need to urinate. (This situation can also occur in a nonpregnant woman with a pelvic mass or with fibroids — masses of fibrous and muscular tissue — in the wall of the uterus. Depending on their location, the fi-

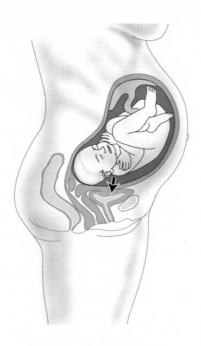

Figure 6. The pregnant uterus
pressing on the bladder

broids can put pressure on the bladder. If you aren't pregnant and find that you must urinate frequently, consult a doctor.)

In addition to the normal reaction of the bladder during pregnancy, there are some effects of pregnancy and childbirth that may lead to incontinence during the pregnancy and immediately after the delivery. Usually, though, the incontinence is temporary and resolves within three to six months of delivery. Many women who develop persistent incontinence after pregnancy either had incontinence symptoms before pregnancy or developed incontinence unrelated to pregnancy. Nonetheless, there are factors, especially during childbirth, that increase the risk of incontinence later in life. About one in five women with stress incontinence developed it in conjunction with pregnancy and delivery. The first vaginal delivery is the single most important event in changing the pelvic-floor structures and in setting the stage for possible stress incontinence in the future. Women who continue to experience stress or urge incontinence three months after their first delivery are at high risk of developing either ongoing or recurrent symptoms.

Of the many changes taking place within a pregnant woman's body, one that can contribute to incontinence is the change in hormone levels. During pregnancy, the placenta secretes a hormone called progesterone. Progesterone is a smooth-muscle relaxant and therefore can weaken the muscles that support the urethra and bladder. With weaker muscles, the bladder neck becomes more mobile and less likely to prevent urine leakage. Sometimes, though rarely, a pregnant woman with a uterus in a posterior position (the top of the uterus tilts backward instead of forward) will experience incomplete emptying of the bladder because the uterus presses on the bladder neck, squeezing it against the pubic bone. Pregnancy may cause incontinence or play a role in the development of incontinence in other ways, too, but researchers and practitioners in medicine and science don't yet know about them. Research projects are continually being undertaken to try to learn more about pregnancy's effects on incontinence.

It's no secret that various parts of a woman's body get stretched during childbirth. As the baby moves into and through the birth canal, organs, muscles, and ligaments in the pelvic region all experience some stretching (Figure 7). Nerves that connect to muscles of the pelvic floor and of the pelvic organs become elongated, and the nerve endings can be damaged. The location of the urethra within the pelvis makes it particularly vulnerable to damage during delivery. The use of instruments such as forceps or vacuum extractors during delivery increases the chance of trauma to the perineum (the skin and thick bar of connective tissue between the opening of the vagina and the opening of the anus), the pelvic floor, and the pelvic organs. All the stretching and injury within the pelvic region can affect the mobility of the urethra and its ability to stay closed, the contraction of the urethral sphincter, and the muscular and ligament support to the pelvic structures. Weakened muscles rely on their surrounding connective tissues for support, but increased pressure within the abdomen can cause these supports to fail. Most often, the damage within the pelvic region leads to stress incontinence.

Various factors during delivery, such as the size of the baby, the

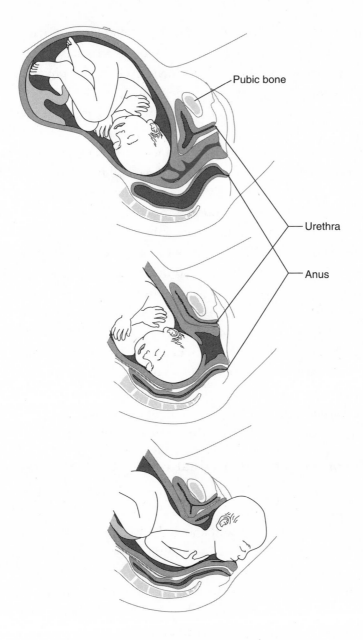

Pubic bone

Urethra

Anus

Figure 7. The effect of pregnancy on the pelvic floor

length of the second stage (the time from full dilation of the cervix to delivery of the entire baby), and the type of anesthesia, may have a role in the development of incontinence. However, physicians continue to debate these factors. At one time, deliveries by cesarean section were thought to protect the pelvic floor and organs from damage during delivery; however, women who undergo cesarean deliveries still have a risk of developing incontinence. This risk stems primarily from the effect of pregnancy itself on the mobility of the bladder neck.

Most women will heal with time, and the changes that occurred during childbirth revert to normal. Sometimes, though, the injuries don't fully heal, and especially with subsequent pregnancies, they result in incontinence. There is some evidence to suggest that training the pelvic-floor muscles before and during pregnancy, and reeducating them after pregnancy, can prevent or improve minor stress incontinence. Pelvic muscle exercises are described in Chapter 6, which discusses nonsurgical treatments for incontinence. Several other factors, including smoking and alcohol intake, also affect a person's predisposition to urinary incontinence. Therefore, if you are considering pregnancy, it is important to ensure an optimal lifestyle, both to maximize the health of the baby and to minimize the risk of developing incontinence during and after the pregnancy and delivery.

## Incontinence with Vaginal Prolapse and Relaxation

The vagina occupies a central position within the pelvic area. In front of the vagina, toward the navel, are the urethra and bladder; behind the vagina is the rectum; and above the vagina is the small intestine, or small bowel. The uterus is a continuation of the vagina via the cervix. The muscles, ligaments, and other tissues that hold the vagina in place contribute to the support of the surrounding pelvic organs. If the vagina's support weakens, the vagina relaxes, and then one or more of the other pelvic organs can also lose support and slip out of position. When an organ is displaced like this, it protrudes into the vagina and is called *prolapse*. The type of prolapse and its severity dictate how the urinary system is affected.

When the front or sides of the vagina lose support, the urethra or bladder, or both, can fall toward and bulge into the vaginal wall

(Figure 8). If only the urethra is involved, the term used is *urethro-cele;* if only the bladder, *cystocele;* and if both are involved — which is the most common type of prolapse in women — *cystourethrocele.*

A urethrocele can be felt as a small bulge at the front part of the entrance to the vagina, but it is rarely a source of discomfort. Sometimes, a woman feels a bulge like this, but it can only be a small cyst or an outpouching of the wall of the urethra. In either of these situations, the bulge occasionally becomes tender. If a urethrocele protrudes outside the vagina, which usually happens along with a cystocele, the woman will feel as if something is hanging out of her. Occasionally, urethrocele is also associated with recurrent bladder or urinary tract infections. If a woman experiences a urethrocele, she won't necessarily experience a cystocele later, though it is always a possibility.

With cystocele, the sagging of the bladder often causes a kink at the bladder neck, where the urethra meets the bladder. This kinking interferes with the ability of the bladder to empty easily and completely. The situation can lead to the feeling of a constant urge to urinate because the bladder retains some urine and therefore continues to give the sensation that it needs to be emptied. The bladder itself usually maintains its muscle tone in the early stages of cystocele, so it can still be possible to completely empty the bladder because of the strength of bladder contractions. However, at later stages, the bladder muscles are often stretched out and lose their ability to overcome the obstructive effect of the kinked bladder neck. It then becomes more and more difficult to completely empty the bladder. In early stages of cystocele, a woman may feel nothing or may at times report a sensation of fullness in the vagina; later on, the vagina may protrude through the vaginal opening.

When support behind the vagina becomes weak, the rectum can protrude into the vagina, termed *rectocele*. Generally, a rectocele results from a defective or weakened vaginal wall or a poorly healed episiotomy. (An episiotomy is an incision made in the perineum to widen the vaginal opening during childbirth.) When a rectocele occurs, the rectum — especially when full — can affect the bladder's ability to function properly because it can press on the bladder neck and

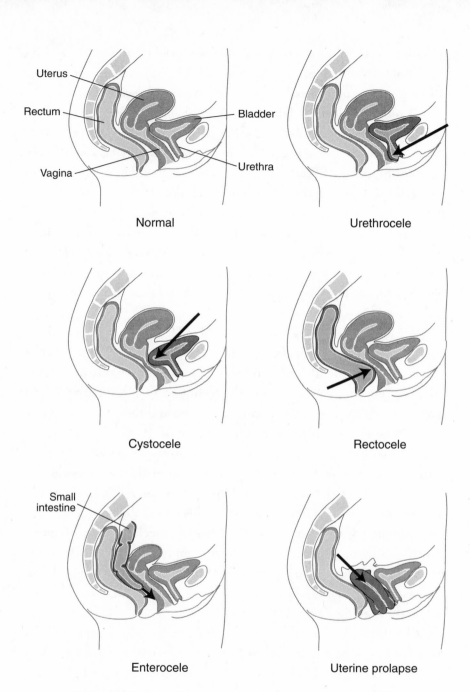

Figure 8. The different types of vaginal prolapse

interfere with urination. The rectocele causes a bulge in the vagina and difficulty in evacuating the rectum. Straining worsens the situation, as it pushes feces into the pouch of the rectum protruding into the vagina. Straining also contributes to weakening of the support structures within the pelvic area.

A weakening of support around the upper and back part of the vagina can result in the small bowel slipping out of position, an *enterocele.* In this instance, the small bowel slips between the vagina and the rectum and generally causes a sensation of pressure and aching in the lower back. An enterocele can interfere with the ability to completely empty the rectum, and as with a rectocele, this difficulty usually leads to straining that further weakens the muscles and ligaments within the pelvis.

Uterine prolapse occurs when the uterus descends into the vagina. The severity of uterine prolapse varies from the cervix sticking through the vaginal opening to the entire uterus protruding outside the vagina. In the case of the cervix protruding, a woman may feel a sensation of heaviness and be able to feel the tip of the cervix with her finger at the entrance of the vagina. For women who have had a hysterectomy (surgical removal of the uterus), the vaginal vault may prolapse. This means that the top of the vagina falls back in on itself, usually because the vagina is in direct contact with the small bowel after the uterus has been removed. Often, an enterocele occurs at the same time as a vaginal vault prolapse.

With any one of the situations of pelvic organ prolapse we have outlined here, the vagina and the supporting muscles and tissues around it are affected, usually relaxing the vagina and making it more mobile. The vagina's mobility plays a role in stress incontinence because when the vagina moves, it displaces the bladder and weakens the urethra's support. The vagina will typically move when abdominal pressure increases as a result of sneezing, coughing, or any of the other activities mentioned earlier. If the urethra itself and the urethral sphincter are still strong, the woman may not experience any incontinence when the vagina moves. However, if the urethra weakens from a loss of muscle mass or from damage to its nerve supply, even a small movement of the vagina could open the urethra (Figure 9).

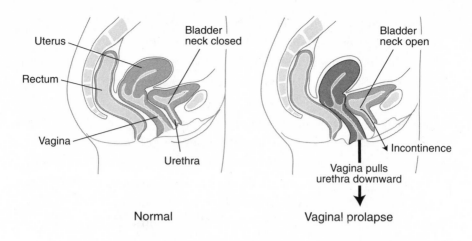

Figure 9. The relationship between urethral weakness and vaginal mobility in causing incontinence

## The Effects of Hysterectomy on Incontinence

A hysterectomy — surgical removal of the uterus — is usually done because of uterine prolapse, excessive bleeding, fibroids (benign tumors in the muscle of the uterus), or malignant tumors. As you recall from earlier descriptions, the uterus is located just above the vagina and behind the bladder. The vagina and bladder share some nerves and surrounding muscle and ligament supports. The greatest potential for a negative effect on the urinary system after a hysterectomy comes from damage to the nerves that extend toward the bladder, since they are detached when the cervix is removed. A carefully performed total or partial hysterectomy should not have any effect on bladder function. A total hysterectomy involves removing the entire uterus and cervix, while a supracervical hysterectomy leaves the cervix intact to help maintain support for the top part of the vagina. Sometimes, though, a woman requires a radical hysterectomy, which is more extensive than removing the uterus alone. In radical hysterectomy, more of the nerve structures may be damaged, resulting in nerve malfunctions that can affect the bladder and urethra and can lead to incontinence and difficulties in urinating. Radical hysterectomy is usually performed to treat cervical cancer and some forms of endometrial cancer involving the cervix. Because the procedure re-

*A Woman's Guide to Urinary Incontinence*

moves so much, it is more likely that nerve damage will occur and result in bladder dysfunction. In addition, a lot of the ligaments of the pelvic region are cut during the operation, which weakens them and affects how well they support the bladder and urethra, leading to incontinence and difficulty in urinating.

Some women will develop incontinence soon after or several years after a hysterectomy. The operation sometimes causes the incontinence, as described above, but not always. In many cases, the pelvic floor and urethral support were already weakened before the hysterectomy, but the uterine symptoms that led to the hysterectomy overshadowed any mild symptoms of bladder dysfunction. The hysterectomy treated the uterine symptoms and left the urinary tract symptoms untreated. Therefore, these urinary tract symptoms are frequently and easily mistaken as the result of the hysterectomy, whereas they probably existed at the outset. For this reason, it is critical to have a complete evaluation of bladder function before proceeding with any type of pelvic surgery; we discuss this and similar issues in Chapter 8, on selecting treatment.

Following difficult hysterectomies and radical hysterectomies, particularly if radiation had already weakened the tissues, poor healing and breakdown of tissues may result in a fistula. A fistula, in which the bladder and vagina are connected, causes continuous leakage of urine through the vagina. Fistulas rarely occur and can be further minimized by prolonged drainage of the bladder with a Foley catheter after a difficult hysterectomy. The repair of fistulas is discussed in Chapter 9, on treatment complications.

## Incontinence during and after Menopause

Menopause occurs when the ovaries stop maturing and releasing eggs, the body produces less of the hormones estrogen and progesterone, and menstruation becomes less frequent and eventually stops. Menopause usually happens between ages 45 and 55, although some women go through an early menopause as young as 35 to 40. For most women, the transition period of menopause lasts for one and a half to two years, and once it's completed, the postmenopausal woman can no longer get pregnant.

The menopause symptom most related to continence is the change in hormone levels in the body, particularly the level of estrogen. The ovaries produce estrogen, so as they become less functional, their production of estrogen declines. The reduced levels of estrogen affect several aspects of the urinary tract. Estrogen maintains the inner linings of the urethra and the bladder, so as estrogen declines, these linings progressively atrophy (lose some mass) and become thinner. This thinning increases the bladder's sensitivity and leads to symptoms of bladder irritability including urgency, frequency, and nocturia. The inner linings of the urethra and the bladder may also become so thin that the tight sealing effect that closes the bladder neck becomes inefficient. This loss of a tight seal favors the development of mixed incontinence, which includes both stress and urge symptoms. Estrogen also promotes blood flow to the pelvic muscles, helping to keep them strong. With less estrogen in the body, the pelvic muscles become weaker, and support for pelvic organs decreases. Muscles such as the urethral sphincter also lose some of their mass and become less efficient at contracting.

Women who undergo surgical removal of their ovaries experience a sudden decline in estrogen, but the effect of the loss of estrogen is slow. Estrogen replacement therapy can be used in a young woman undergoing premenopausal removal of the ovaries. In addition to maintaining estrogen levels, estrogen replacement seems to improve the bladder's ability to prevent infections.

## The Effects of Diabetes and Metabolic Diseases on Incontinence

Diabetes mellitus, commonly referred to as diabetes, is a disease in which the body doesn't produce enough insulin or doesn't use insulin efficiently, resulting in high glucose, or sugar, levels in the blood and urine. The disease affects the function of small nerves and blood vessels. It also affects the bladder in several ways. When diabetes first develops, or if it is out of control, the body often produces large amounts of urine. The person may experience this as frequent urination, often with urgency, and she may wake up frequently at night to urinate. A woman with advanced or severe diabetes often has reduced bladder sensation, and the bladder may empty only partially or even completely retain urine when she tries to urinate. If the urethral sphincter is weak, there may be overflow incontinence.

Diabetes also affects the ability of tissues to heal after surgery, and the tissues are at greater risk of infection in the presence of foreign materials, which may be implanted during surgery (see Chapter 7 for details on surgical treatments). Thus, diabetic women may have fewer treatment options, or they may experience greater complication rates than women who do not have diabetes.

Nondiabetic people who take diuretic medications ("water pills") for high blood pressure or other reasons may experience a similar effect on the bladder — urge and overflow incontinence — in the hours shortly after taking their medication when urine output is increased. The symptoms then subside until the medication is taken again.

## Incontinence in People with Neurological Injury or Illness

Because the bladder and urethral sphincter are under the control of the central nervous system, diseases and injuries that affect any part of the nervous system can affect bladder function and urinary control. It is unusual for incontinence to be the first symptom to indicate that a person has a neurological disease, but it does happen. For example, incontinence is the first symptom to appear for about 10 percent of people subsequently diagnosed with multiple sclerosis, and incontinence may be the only symptom of spinal cord tumors and spinal stenosis (constriction of the spinal cord nerves by arthritic thickening of the bones and ligaments around them). Thus, if unusual incontinence appears in a young woman who has previously been healthy, the woman should be evaluated for a newly developed neurological disease. Caught early, some neurological conditions respond well to treatment.

### Stroke, Brain Injury, and Brain Tumor

The brain is a critical structure in the control of bladder function (Figure 10). The brain is the part of the body where signals coming from the bladder become conscious, and it is also the part of the body

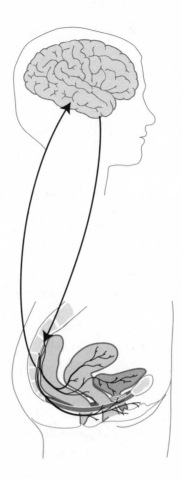

Figure 10. The relationship of the
brain to the urinary tract

where voluntary signals controlling the bladder originate. Therefore,
a stroke or a brain tumor can significantly affect bladder control.

A stroke occurs when part of the brain is deprived of its blood supply, either through narrowed or hardened arteries or through a temporary blockage from a blood clot (embolus). The damaged area can
no longer function to originate or conduct signals. People who have
had a stroke have a difficult time controlling their bladder contractions because the bladder is no longer regulated by the brain. Thus,
the bladder behaves much like a newborn's bladder: it fills to a cer-

*A Woman's Guide to Urinary Incontinence*

tain point, and then a reflex contraction starts. The sphincter voluntarily relaxes, and the bladder contracts and expels the urine it contains. A person who has had a stroke may have some awareness of urgency or a sense that urine is passing but cannot be stopped. She may also make frequent trips to the toilet but have difficulty in starting the urine flow. Depending on the severity and permanence of the stroke injury, this combination of reflex contraction and difficulty in urinating will usually dominate over other contributing causes of incontinence.

The patterns of bladder dysfunction and incontinence resulting from brain injuries and brain tumors are less specific than those resulting from strokes. The location of the injury or the tumor determines the effect on bladder control, though often the problem is similar to that seen after a stroke. The common features of incontinence for people with a brain injury or tumor are a loss of awareness of bladder events, involuntary contractions of the bladder, or incomplete contractions of the bladder leading to more frequent urination.

## Spinal Cord Injury

The spinal cord transmits signals between the brain and the bladder, and it coordinates the contraction and relaxation of the bladder and the urethral sphincter. Thus, spinal cord injuries — whether partial or complete, whether affecting the upper or lower cord — can result in dramatic changes in bladder function and continence.

When the spinal cord is damaged above the waist (cervical or thoracic), the bladder can develop powerful spasms that expel urine at unpredictable and undesirable times. Sometimes only some of the urine in the bladder is expelled, and at other times the bladder is completely emptied by one of these spasms. These spasms are often associated with simultaneous contractions of the urethral sphincter, which tries to block passage along the urethra. When the sphincter contracts like this, the bladder is acting against a strong obstruction. The concern in this case is that urine reflux, or backflow of urine into the kidneys, will occur and cause kidney damage.

When the cord is damaged below the waist (lumbar or sacral), the urethral sphincter becomes partially paralyzed, and the bladder becomes floppy, contracts poorly or not at all, and in later phases may become stiff and resistant to expansion. There will often be a loss of sensation not only in the bladder but also in the surrounding area of the buttocks and genitals, so-called saddle anesthesia. This kind of lower-cord injury may be limited to the bladder and the rectum and may completely spare the legs. In other words, someone with a lower-cord injury may be able to walk but could still have paralysis in some pelvic regions. The bladder may simply overflow without the woman having any awareness that it was full. The amount of leakage will depend almost entirely on how much function or muscle mass the urethral sphincter has. This kind of overflow problem causes symptoms much like those of simple stress incontinence, but because of the associated bladder injury, it does not often respond to the conventional treatments for stress incontinence (discussed in Chapters 6 and 7).

### Spina Bifida

Spina bifida is a relatively rare but fairly well recognized birth defect that affects the development of the spinal cord. With rare exception, it is diagnosed in childhood. Most spina bifida conditions usually affect the lower spine, and the incontinence problems that result are similar to those in women with lower spinal cord injuries.

Women with spina bifida who develop urinary incontinence later in life have a much more complex problem than other women with incontinence. Not only must the causes of the incontinence be identified, but also the bladder changes associated with spina bifida must be considered. For example, there may be changes in sensation, capacity, compliance, or contractility, and there may be a loss of normal urethral resistance or coordination.

A mild form of spina bifida is the absence of the sacral bone — a broad, flat bone at the bottom of the spinal column. The nerves to the bladder and the urethral sphincter travel through small openings in this bone. The absence of the sacral bone is often associated with abnormal function of, damage to, or inadequate development of these nerves. This condition, called sacral agenesis, is often subtle, as it may affect only the nerves to the bladder and the rectum. In fact, in a woman who has this condition, it may be discovered only when she is examined for stress incontinence. A simple X-ray of the pelvis is enough to show the absence of the sacral bone, but magnetic resonance imaging (MRI) or other testing may be required to identify important details.

### Spinal Stenosis

Spinal stenosis is a condition that affects people as they age. The bones and ligaments thicken because of arthritis, and the spinal cord or its nerves become trapped by the growth of the spine. The majority of people with this condition usually first notice pain or numbness affecting the legs or buttocks. Sometimes, a subtle, early sign is a loss of the sensation that the bladder is filling. In most women, this loss of sensation will lead to overstretching of the bladder, decreasing ability to empty the bladder, or urinary retention, which means they try to urinate but can't. In women with a weak urethra, the bladder fullness resulting from decreased sensation may lead to overflow incontinence. Spinal stenosis is not a common cause of bladder dysfunction, but it should be considered when there is diminished sensation of bladder filling and there are no other plausible reasons for this symptom.

### Pelvic Operations and Injuries

Extensive operations on the pelvis, such as radical hysterectomy for cancer of the cervix or the uterus, can affect the nerves to the bladder. The damage most commonly sustained is loss of sensation as the bladder fills. This is usually associated with partial or complete retention of urine in the bladder when the woman attempts to urinate. When the urethra is weak, however, overflow incontinence can result as the distended bladder overcomes the limited resistance of the weakened urethra. In addition, a fistula, or connection, can form between the bladder or urethra and the vagina, resulting in continuous leakage of urine. Fistulas are most likely to form after extensive dissection of ligaments and other tissues, especially with multiple surgeries, and after radiation treatment, which can contribute to poor healing and breakdown of tissues. Fistulas can occur from the trauma to the pelvic area when a woman goes through obstructed labor that isn't eased by a cesarean section. Finally, fistulas may also form after an accident that causes trauma to the pelvic region and breaks down the natural barriers between organs.

## Parkinson Disease

Parkinson disease is a common disease of older and occasionally younger people. It is a slowly progressing, degenerative disorder of the nervous system that results in tremor, rigidity, and impaired muscle control. As a result of the nerve damage, people with Parkinson disease develop urgency and urge incontinence, which is generally treated by medication to reduce sudden bladder contractions and minimize urgency.

## Multiple Sclerosis

Multiple sclerosis is a slowly progressive neurological disease that usually affects young women (and men). It diminishes the protective sheath, called myelin, that covers the larger, longer nerves in the body and serves as an insulator in the brain. The loss of myelin interferes with nerve pathways and causes muscles to gradually become weaker. Over time, people with this disease lose the coordination and function of organs that rely on the affected nerves. About 10 percent of people with multiple sclerosis have bladder symptoms in early stages of the disease, but as many as 90 percent will have them as the disease reaches a more advanced stage. Multiple sclerosis causes a gradual separation of the bladder from brain control, and the coordination of the bladder and the urethral sphincter deteriorates. The typical symptoms are urgency, frequency, urge incontinence, and partial emptying of the bladder. Sometimes there is also stress incontinence, but urgency is usually the dominant problem.

## Enuresis

Enuresis, or bedwetting, is usually thought to be a problem limited to childhood, something a person simply outgrows. Indeed, almost all children who wet the bed stop doing so by age 5. Nevertheless, there are an estimated 7 million adult bedwetters in the world. The problem for most adult bedwetters is thought to be neurological, a problem in specialized centers in the brain that are unable to sense signals from the bladder warning of the need to urinate. It may be more complex than just "deep sleeping." Usually, an adult with enuresis has normal daytime bladder control.

## The Effects of Aging on Incontinence

Aging causes changes within the body that affect all levels of bladder function. These changes include a lack of estrogen, weakening of connective tissue and muscles, and diminished function of nerves. Changes in other organ systems also influence how the bladder functions. For example, kidney function changes with age, usually with the kidneys working better at night than during the day. The increased kidney function at night often results from blood vessels becoming less efficient at returning blood to the heart, allowing blood to pool in the legs during the day. The pooled fluid usually shifts in the body at night, and the kidneys process the fluid, thus increasing the output of urine. Therefore, an older woman often finds herself getting up at night to empty her bladder, a condition called nocturia.

As described in the section on menopause, low estrogen levels cause the lining of the urethra to become thinner, to the point that the urethra often loses its ability to remain tightly closed. Blood flow to the pelvic region decreases, too, and reduces even further the sealing effect of the urethra. The bladder's lining also becomes thinner and hence becomes more sensitive to urine stored in the bladder. With less estrogen in the body, the bladder and urethral muscles themselves atrophy, or lose some mass, making the muscles less efficient at contracting. In fact, the volume of muscle cells and fibers in the urethra and urethral sphincter begins to decrease early in childhood and continues to decrease with age. With less mass, the striated muscle of the urethral sphincter becomes less effective during episodes of physical stress, and so the backup mechanism for the urethra begins to fail and allows urine to leak out.

With age, the connective tissues that support the urethra and pelvic organs become less elastic. Changes in the support of the pelvic organs and pelvic floor put additional strain on the bladder and bladder neck and contribute to weakening the urethral sphincter. When the urethra is easily displaced because of poor support, the function of the urethral sphincter can also be altered by the lack of support. These changes in connective tissue supports result in symptoms of stress incontinence.

The delicate nerve system throughout the urinary tract becomes progressively slower over time at conducting information to the pelvic organs and other structures. The organs and structures become less responsive to the signals they receive, and they also respond less often because they receive fewer signals. The reduced nerve function means that for older women a larger volume of urine may remain in the bladder after urination and the bladder's capacity becomes functionally smaller. An older woman also has a reduced perception of bladder fullness that delays the urge to urinate when the bladder is excessively full, leading to overflow incontinence. In addition, changes in nerve function can increase the bladder muscle's activity and lead to premature contractions, thus decreasing the bladder's ability to store urine.

Chronic lung disorders that cause a person to cough frequently will stretch and weaken the urethral sphincter, eventually leading to its failure. Chronic constipation also causes weakening of the urethral sphincter through repeated straining. The effects of these chronic conditions slowly accumulate over time.

Older women are more likely to develop other conditions that can affect their bladder function. For example, they are more likely to contract urinary tract infections. The irritation from such an infection can overcome the normal control mechanisms and result in incontinence that remains until the infection is treated. Older women also have a tendency to develop diabetes, which results in increased urinary output, as described earlier, as well as neural dysfunction that can lead to incontinence.

Reflexes gradually slow down as people age. The tightening of the urethral sphincter is a reflex that attempts to stop or prevent a bladder contraction. When a normal or strong urge to urinate develops, an older person may lack the quickness of response to stop the bladder contraction that follows the urge.

Finally, very elderly people may have problems of dementia or reduced mental awareness of body functions and surroundings. In these circumstances, a woman can lose awareness of the bladder, with resulting overflow incontinence or bladder overactivity.

## Other Circumstances That Cause or Affect Incontinence

A number of other circumstances can affect the proper function of the urinary system. For example, obesity, smoking, and ingestion of bladder irritants including alcohol, coffee, and acid-promoting substances may overwhelm a bladder that functions at only a borderline level. Also, radiation therapy can cause scarring of the bladder, which leads to smaller capacity and irritability. Finally, a person who is unable to move fast enough when urgency develops may experience functional incontinence — the inability to make it to the toilet on time. In this situation, a bedside commode can help to alleviate the problem.

With a general understanding of the urinary tract system and incontinence, you probably already have some idea of the type of incontinence you are experiencing. Armed with this information and knowing some of the terms used, you are now in an excellent position to consult a doctor for a medical evaluation, as discussed in the next chapter.

# Consulting a Doctor: How to Find
# the Right Physician and What You Can Expect

Some women will find ways to cope with urinary incontinence for several years before seeking a doctor's help, while other women will decide to consult a physician as soon as they realize they may have a problem. Only you can decide when the right time has arrived for you to go to a doctor. Whether you want to consult a physician immediately or wait for a while, it will help you to have some information about finding a doctor, what a doctor's visit will entail, and how a doctor will assess you. In this chapter, we begin by describing how to find a doctor and the types of doctor you may encounter. We continue with details about what to expect during the first appointment and how to prepare for it so you can provide the doctor with as much helpful information as possible and also get answers to your questions. We then describe how the doctor conducts the physical examination. The chapter closes with a section about assessing your situation so that you and the physician can decide what steps to take next.

## Finding the Right Doctor

Your primary-care physician is the doctor you will most likely consult first when you decide to seek help for urinary incontinence. A primary-care physician can be a family doctor, an internist, or a geriatrician who has been caring for your general health or an allied health care professional such as a physician assistant, nurse, or nurse practitioner. In the initial phase of incontinence, when you recognize it merely as a nuisance, your primary-care physician can evaluate whether you have a urinary tract infection, one common cause of incontinence. A urinary tract infection can be treated with antibiotics. While they can increase urgency and may worsen an underlying incontinence condition, urinary tract infections don't generally predispose a woman to future incontinence.

If an infection is ruled out, the next step involves evaluating your medical history as it relates to the urinary tract and bladder, a physical examination, and possibly diagnostic testing. Some primary-care physicians will conduct this evaluation themselves, but many will give you a referral to see a specialist, usually a urologist or a gynecologist and sometimes a colorectal surgeon. A urologist specializes in disorders of the urinary tract, from the kidneys to the urethra. Some urologists have a specific interest in female urinary incontinence as part of a larger interest in both male and female incontinence and voiding dysfunction. A gynecologist specializes in the function and disorders of the reproductive tract, including pregnancy and its effect on the pelvic floor as well as the urogenital organs. You may also come across a urogynecologist, a physician who focuses on problems of urinary incontinence specifically related to obstetrics and gynecology. A colorectal surgeon's primary interest is the lower bowel tract. Ask your primary-care physician about the particular interests and experience of the specialist to whom you are being referred.

Frequently, a woman requires the input of several physicians with different specialties to determine the cause of urinary incontinence and the best way to treat it. In addition to the specialists mentioned above, you may be referred to one or more of the following:

- A gastroenterologist, who specializes in diseases of the digestive tract including anorectal function and incontinence
- A neurologist, who specializes in diseases of the nervous system, several of which can alter bladder and urethral function and cause incontinence

- A physical therapist, who helps you recover some of the function of your pelvic muscle to aid with pelvic-floor support and reinforcement of urinary control

If you are referred to some of these experts, you may see them only once or twice, but their input can be critical in providing a good long-term result in your situation.

When you go to your primary-care physician, you may feel embarrassed to describe some of the problems you're having. It's not easy to talk about personal health issues, particularly when they are as private as incontinence. However, the more information and details you can provide your physician, the more likely it is that you will get a referral to the most appropriate specialist.

*Ginny began noticing episodes in which a small amount of urine leaked out when she played soccer. She was a forward on the local women's team, which competed in a regional league. She had joined the team four years earlier, and she loved the twice weekly practices, as much for the exercise as for the friendships. She didn't think too much of the leaking at first because she also sweated a lot during soccer practice, but the volume gradually increased, and she began using pads to soak it up. The incontinence continued to get worse, and Ginny started making excuses not to attend the soccer practices and games. A few months later, she had an appointment for a routine Pap smear and thought that perhaps she should mention the leaking to her doctor. She was so embarrassed, though, that she didn't bring it up. Afterward, she was annoyed and frustrated with herself and resolved to make another appointment. She waffled for weeks, picking up the phone and putting it back down. What would her doctor's reaction be? And what could he really do to help her? Finally, she called and booked an appointment. Her nervousness was apparent when the doctor came into the consulting room, but Ginny managed to describe the situation. Her doctor acted as though he heard this problem described every day. He asked her several questions and then suggested that he refer her to a local urologist. Ginny was relieved that she had finally broached the topic, and she felt more in control now that she was taking some positive steps toward resolving her problem.*

In the case example above, Ginny need not have feared an uncaring reaction from her doctor. In most instances, physicians will listen to your concerns and take them seriously. Unfortunately, though, a few doctors will not be as attentive as they should be and may even dismiss your concerns. In the past, many doctors considered incontinence to be simply an inconvenience or a natural part of aging, rather than a significant health issue. Thanks to better information and understanding, incontinence is slowly being acknowledged by more and more health care professionals as the health concern that it is. If your family doctor, or even the specialist you've been referred to, doesn't take your situation as seriously as you wish, then consider finding a different doctor. Ask friends or family for recommendations, look at the listings in the yellow pages, or contact an organization such as the National Association for Continence (see the Resources section at the end of the book) for a list of specialists in your area. Ultimately, you need to find a doctor who is knowledgeable about and sympathetic to the type of problem you are experiencing and with whom you feel comfortable discussing your situation.

At the end of this book, we list resources to help you identify physicians with specific interest in problems related to the urinary tract, pelvic floor, and pelvic organs.

## Becoming a Partner in Your Health Care

The relationship you have with your doctor affects the decisions you make and the outcome of any treatments you undergo. Your doctor will give you information and make suggestions and recommendations based on his or her knowledge and experience, but you are ultimately the person who should decide how you want to proceed. If you are an active partner in deciding how to address the problem you're dealing with, you will maintain control over your situation. You can do several things to be an effective partner in your health care:

- Find out as much as you can about the problem you're having. Reading this book is a great first step. You might also find information on the Internet, in publications by incontinence organizations, or through a support group. Some places to find additional information are listed in the Resources section at the end of the book.

- Tell the doctor at your first appointment that you want to be involved in making decisions about diagnostic tests and treatment options. He or she will almost certainly be happy and encouraged that you want to play an active part in your health care. If your wish is not respected, consider finding a different doctor.

- Be open and forthcoming about the symptoms you experience, previous treatments you've tried (if any), and the expectations you have. The doctor will be able to help you most by knowing everything relevant to your situation.

- Prepare for your appointments by writing a list of questions you want answered. Later in the chapter, we suggest questions you may want to ask. If the doctor uses terms you don't understand to explain the diagnosis and treatment options, ask more questions.

- Take notes during or after the appointment with your doctor. If you get distracted by writing notes, ask for a copy of the doctor's consultation notes or tape-record the appointment. You can also bring someone along to serve as an observer, to help you remember later the events and discussions that took place during the appointment.

## Identifying the Best Approach for You

When you've made the decision to consult a doctor or you have a referral to a specialist, think about whether you want to go to the appointment by yourself or with someone else. Some people prefer to see a doctor alone, but it is perfectly acceptable to take someone with you to the consultation. Some women, for example, become nervous or flustered, forget things easily, or feel intimidated when they're in a doctor's office, so taking someone to the appointment helps to ensure that the discussion is as productive as possible. You may decide to ask your spouse, a close friend, a relative, or a mature child to accompany you and provide support during or after the consultation. There may be times when you prefer to consult with the doctor by yourself, times when you want to have someone accompany you, and times when you wish to discuss your problems with someone else but still go alone to the doctor. All these approaches are valid.

Also keep in mind that you don't have to be in a hurry to make decisions about options or treatments. Proceed at your own pace and be comfortable with your understanding of the information you receive from the doctor. In fact, we recommend that you take time to consider the information and options your physician provides before deciding on your next step. It can be easy to focus solely on the most optimistic outcome the doctor describes without assessing both the advantages and disadvantages of a particular treatment.

## What to Expect from Your First Appointment with a Specialist

The first appointment you have with a gynecologist or urologist can be quite detailed and can take from 30 minutes to an hour. The doctor will begin by asking you questions about your medical history and experiences with incontinence. Some doctors give you a printed questionnaire to fill out ahead of time and then ask you for further details during the appointment. The physician asks a wide range of questions to gather information about past surgeries and hospitalizations, pregnancies, medications, drug allergies, lifestyle, and family history of problems. He or she will then ask specific questions to find out about

- your bladder function, including difficulty with starting to urinate, discomfort while urinating, hesitancy or interruption of urine flow, and feeling like the bladder is not completely emptied;
- your digestive tract and how well it functions, particularly the colon and rectum, because this information helps to evaluate the functioning of the pelvic floor;
- any instances of blood in the urine, kidney stones, tumors, or injuries, including operations, head and spine injuries, and car accidents;
- the nature of your incontinence, such as when it occurs, how

much leakage you have, what activity you are doing at the time, and whether you get any warning that leakage will occur;

- the severity of your incontinence — for example, the number of panties or pads you use in a day;
- the limitations incontinence causes in your social and professional life, such as avoiding friends or not attending social activities; and
- any evaluations and treatments you've already undertaken and their results, as well as how the incontinence has changed over time.

Some of the questions the doctor asks you will seem awkward to answer, and others will be flat-out embarrassing. Remember, though, that the doctor has heard answers to these questions many times before and will not be embarrassed by any of your descriptions. Try to be as direct and specific as possible in your responses, and clarify or expand on previous answers if something else occurs to you later in the discussion.

After taking down your history, the doctor will then conduct a physical examination and may order additional medical tests to help in making a diagnosis. The most common test is a urine analysis, or urinalysis, which is described in detail, along with other tests, in Chapter 5. Before discussing these parts of the appointment, however, it is helpful to find out how to best prepare for your appointment.

## Preparing for Your Appointment

You will get the most out of your appointment if you go prepared with the information the doctor needs to help make a diagnosis and with the questions you want answered. It can also be helpful to think about your expectations and goals before you see the doctor. Write them down, if this helps you determine what they are. By having a clear idea of what you want to find out from consulting the doctor, you will be in a better position to assess the information he or she gives you and to decide what steps you want to take next.

Most of the doctor's questions during the appointment will be about your bladder function and the severity of incontinence that you experience. So that you can accurately answer these questions, keep a bladder diary for at least three days and ideally for a week. Record all relevant events:

- The amount and type of fluid you consume each day. Fluid includes all liquid drinks and also liquid foods, such as soup.
- The amount of urine you pass when you use the toilet, the time of day (or night), and whether you had the urge to go at the time.
- How much urine comes out during accidental leaks and what you were doing at the time (e.g., sneezing, exercising, lifting a heavy object, having sex).
- The number of pads you use during the day or the number of times you change panties.
- The circumstances of nighttime leakage, including whether you wake up with an urge to urinate or already wet, whether you can make it to the toilet or you leak on the way, and how much leakage you have and at what times it occurs, if you know.

A bladder diary helps you and the doctor recognize whether your incontinence is related to physical activity, the urge to urinate, or both, or possibly to drinking too much fluid or producing too much urine. A sample diary page is shown in Figure 11.

Before going to your appointment, try to remember the dates and circumstances when you first realized that you might have a problem with urinary incontinence. The initiating circumstances often suggest the most likely cause of incontinence. Some women can recall a precise event, while for others there was a less well-defined moment.

*Pattie, for example, clearly recalls attending a conference banquet in a hotel when she suddenly and quite unexpectedly lost control of her bladder. Her panties were wet, and, fearing that the moisture would soak through to the outside of her skirt, she quickly excused herself from the table and fled to her hotel room. Fortunately, the urine was not visible on her skirt, and she changed and returned to the banquet. She was nonetheless embarrassed and confused about the accidental leak.*

| DATE: | | NAME: | | | |
|---|---|---|---|---|---|
| TIME | DRINKS | URINE | URGE | LEAKS | TYPE OF ACTIVITY |
| 00:00 am/pm | # Ounces | # Ounces | Y / N | S / M / L | Laughing, lifting, etc. |
| | | | | | |
| | | | | | |
| 8A | 12 | | | | Breakfast |
| 9A | | 10 | N | N | Resting |
| 11A | | 2 | Y | M | Shopping |
| 2P | | 3 | N | L | Exercise |
| 4P | 12 | | | | Tea |
| | | | | | |
| | | | | | |
| | | | | | |
| | | | | | |
| | | | | | |
| | | | | | |
| | | | | | |
| | | | | | |
| | | | | | |
| | | | | | |
| | | | | | |
| | | | | | |
| | | | | | |
| | | | | | |
| | | | | | |
| | | | | | |
| | | | | | |
| TOTALS | | | | | |

Figure 11. Bladder diary

*Heather began noticing during her first pregnancy that she occasionally leaked urine, but she couldn't pinpoint a specific time or event when she first noticed it. As her pregnancy progressed, she found that she leaked more often and that more fluid escaped. After she delivered her baby, the leaking persisted. The incontinence both annoyed and embarrassed her, especially when she took her baby to mom-and-tot groups and the other mothers didn't seem to have this problem.*

It is also helpful to take copies of records you have from previous evaluations and treatments as well as reports from operations. Sometimes your records will be forwarded when a referral is made, but often you will have to make the request yourself. If you take any medications, make a list of them with details including the name of the drug, the dose you take, and how frequently you take it. Finally, if you have noticed any circumstances that appear to alleviate your incontinence, such as altering your diet or lifestyle, make a note of them to tell the doctor.

## Questions to Ask the Doctor

You've been reading about urinary incontinence in this book and perhaps elsewhere, and you may have heard some information on the radio or television or from other people. Before you go to your appointment, therefore, you have some idea of what you want to find out from the doctor. So that you leave the doctor's office with all the information you want, prepare a list of questions beforehand. While the doctor is answering your questions, make notes, or ask a person accompanying you to make notes.

Your list of questions may include some of the following, as well as others that are more specific to your situation. You will also find more information to help answer some of the questions below in later chapters of this book. The doctor may be able to answer only some of these questions after an initial consultation, while others will have to wait for a more detailed assessment.

What type of incontinence do I have?
What are the causes of my incontinence?

What are the diagnostic tests that you are ordering and why?

When will you have a diagnosis?

What are the treatment options? Are there any other options?

What are the advantages and disadvantages of the recommended treatment?

Are there any risks or complications from the recommended treatment?

How much will the treatment cost?

Will the treatment require hospitalization? How long will it take to resume normal activities?

Will the treatment completely eliminate the incontinence I currently experience?

## What to Expect during the Physical Examination

The physical examination gives your doctor several clues about what may be causing your incontinence. You will be asked to change into a hospital gown in a private room, and the doctor will then examine you to determine whether you have any conditions that might affect the function of your urinary tract. Most often, the doctor will first assess your general health by taking some basic measurements, such as blood pressure, pulse, temperature, and respiratory rate. Next, the doctor assesses your nervous system, which is responsible for muscle function, perception, reflexes, and conscious awareness. The nervous system testing may include moving limbs, looking at the back, testing the response to a pinprick or to a light touch with something like a cotton swab, and testing reflexes with a reflex hammer. Some of the areas involved may be around the pubic area or the rectum, since these skin areas reflect changes that occur in the parts of the nervous system affecting the bladder.

The doctor will then ask you to lie on your back with your legs bent at the knees and your feet supported by stirrups so he or she can examine your abdomen, pelvis, and rectum. This part of the physical examination may feel a little uncomfortable, but it should not be painful when performed by a skilled examiner. If it is, tell your doctor.

The abdominal examination takes a few minutes. The doctor looks at and may tap or press on various parts of the abdomen to feel your bladder and other organs and determine if anything is enlarged, tender, or abnormal.

The pelvic examination is similar to a regular gynecology exam, with an additional first step to look at the skin between the vagina and anus (called the perineum) and to determine the strength of the pelvic-floor muscles in this area. A visual inspection of the perineum provides clues about the degree of irritation from constant moisture, the position of the anus relative to the vagina, and the condition of the circular muscles around the anus (anal sphincter). Using a cotton swab, the doctor will evaluate the sensation and reflexes of the perineum by gently touching the clitoris and the area around the anus to make the muscles contract. The doctor will then use one or two fingers to assess the tone and reflexes of the pelvic-floor muscles while asking you to bear down, hold back, cough, and strain. He or she will ask you to repeat these actions several times while the lips of the vulva are spread and while the doctor's fingers support different areas around the pelvic floor. The finger support allows other weak areas to be identified. This step allows the doctor to evaluate the position of the pelvic organs and how much they move during stressful events such as coughing or straining. Often when a woman coughs or strains as instructed, there will be some incontinence. Don't be embarrassed: the doctor expects and needs to see urine leakage to determine how and when your incontinence occurs.

When the doctor is ready to examine the vagina and cervix, he or she will insert a speculum, which is a metal or plastic device with two blades that open and hold apart the walls of the vagina. To determine where and how the pelvic organs are supported, the doctor will use the speculum blades to support the front or back of the vagina while you strain. The doctor will then insert one or two gloved fingers into the vagina and press on the abdomen with the other hand to feel for any abnormality behind the uterus, of the urethra, around the bladder, or at the base of the bladder. At this point, the doctor will ask you to contract the pelvic-floor muscles to assess their strength, as well as your ability to recognize and separate these muscles from your abdominal wall and thigh muscles.

The final part of the physical examination is to assess the rectum and anus. The doctor will check the tone and strength of the anal sphincter by inserting a finger into the rectum while asking you to contract the muscles. This assessment allows the doctor to look for any weakness in front of the rectum.

## Assessing Your Situation and Selecting the Next Step

After the medical history and physical examination, your doctor will have the basic information needed to make a diagnosis or pursue further testing. He or she should review the information with you and discuss its relevance to your situation. At this point, the doctor may talk about possible treatment options or may suggest further investigation with one or more diagnostic tests. The decision to proceed with tests or with treatment is yours to make with the assistance and advice of your physician. You may want to take some time to think about the severity of your situation and the degree to which your life is disrupted by incontinence. If you feel able to cope with the incontinence you currently experience, you may decide to wait and proceed with further testing or treatment only if the situation worsens. However, it can often be beneficial to continue with some testing to rule out causes of incontinence that can be immediately and easily corrected before they progress.

A number of simple measures can be instituted whose response can help provide an answer to the question of whether further investigation or treatment should be carried out. For example, as a first step, you may be asked to change your fluid intake habits by drinking less fluid, restricting fluids after 7 p.m., or decreasing your intake of coffee, tea, and caffeinated soft drinks, which can stimulate bladder overactivity. The doctor may also suggest altering your urination habits by increasing the frequency of urination to reduce the chances of unexpected leakage or using certain types of absorbent pads to help in critical times when the risk of incontinence is greatest. Finally, the doctor may review your medications to see whether any of them might be contributing to incontinence; sleeping medications, sedatives and tranquilizers, and diuretics are well-known contributors to incontinence.

The next chapter discusses in detail the various medical tests that your physician may recommend to get a better understanding of your incontinence. Chapters 6 and 7 explain the treatment options available, and Chapter 8 discusses how to select the best treatment in your case.

## ♀ 5 ♀

## *Medical Tests:*

## *Why and How Are They Done?*

After assessing your medical history and the results of the physical examination, your doctor may suggest one or more medical tests to help make a diagnosis or determine the most appropriate treatment in your situation. In this chapter, we describe the tests, including how they are done and what information they provide. We begin with the simple tests, which are urine analysis (urinalysis) and pad weighing, and continue with more complex tests, including assessment of the lower urinary tract (bladder or urodynamic test), visual inspection inside the bladder (cystoscopy), and imaging by X-ray, ultrasound, and magnetic resonance imaging (MRI). The goals of testing are to determine the relative contribution (or role) of bladder function, urethral resistance to leakage, and vaginal support to a single person's specific incontinence.

### Urinalysis

One of the oldest diagnostic tests in medicine is the visual inspection of urine. In medieval times, a physician summoned to the bedside would first send an assistant to obtain a fresh sample of urine from the patient. The physician would hold the urine sample in the daylight and examine its color and clarity; he might smell it and even taste it! This inspection of urine is called uroscopy (not to be confused with cystoscopy, which we describe later in this chapter). Although the diagnostic capabilities of urologists and gynecologists have expanded greatly since the early practice of medicine, the simple urinalysis remains an excellent test of urinary tract health. Urinalysis is particularly helpful in evaluating a woman with incontinence for infection and bleeding and as a simple screening test for other diseases.

When asked to provide a urine sample, a patient receives a small plastic cup or jar and a cleansing wipe or towelette to take into the washroom. A good urine sample will catch part of the midstream of freely flowing urine. It helps to part the lips of the vulva with your fingers, clean the urethral opening with the cleansing wipe, and then allow some urine to flow before collecting the midstream flow in the cup. If you have an empty bladder, the doctor may ask you to drink fluids and wait at the office until you have produced enough urine to give a sample. Some women have "bashful bladders" and find it difficult or impossible to provide a urine sample in an unfamiliar setting. In these instances, the doctor may place a small catheter into the bladder to drain off urine. This procedure is painless and uses sterile equipment to minimize the risk of introducing infection.

A doctor may examine the urine at his or her office or send the sample to a clinical laboratory. Normal urine has a faint but distinctive odor. Foul-smelling urine almost always indicates infection. Normal urine is slightly yellow and clear enough to easily read newsprint through it. Hazy urine may indicate an infection or the presence of protein, while bloody or tea-colored urine signals bleeding from the urinary tract. The presence of blood in the urine must always be investigated further because it may be caused by kidney stones or another serious condition. As well as visually examining the urine, the doctor or technician will dip a special plastic strip into the urine (dipstick test) to reveal the presence of protein, bile, sugar and its by-products, and blood or blood components too small to see with the eye. The dipstick also indicates the acidity of the urine, and some types of dipsticks can detect bacterial by-products suggesting infection. Finally, the doctor or technician examines the urine with a microscope to look for blood cells, pus cells, bacteria, and crystals.

Depending on the results of the urinalysis, a urine sample may be sent to a specialized laboratory to further examine cells that have been shed from the lining of the urinary tract or to determine how many and what kinds of bacteria or fungi are growing in the urine. This information can guide your doctor in prescribing the correct antibiotics for treatment of difficult urinary tract infections.

## Pad-Weighing Test

When you visit a physician to seek help for urinary incontinence, he or she will want to know how much urine you leak. It can be difficult to answer this question accurately, although it's possible to estimate the amount of urine by the size and number of pads you wear during a single day and the length of time you have been using pads.

A more accurate way to estimate the amount of urine lost, and to be able to compare the amount before and after treatment, is to perform a pad-weighing test. A woman is given a standard-size absorbent pad to wear for a short period of time in the doctor's office or for a longer time at home. In the office, the woman may be asked to drink a certain amount of fluid and perform certain movements to provoke urine to seep out. The fluid will be absorbed into the pad, which is then weighed. If you take the pad home to do the test, record the length of time you wear the pad and then seal it inside a plastic bag to return it to the doctor.

## Bladder Test

A bladder test, also known as a urodynamic test, assesses how the urinary tract behaves as the bladder fills up and as it empties again. Together, the filling and emptying complete one bladder cycle. The test results provide valuable information about the urethra's strength and about how the bladder feels, how much it holds, and how much pressure urine puts on it, all of which help in diagnosing the cause of incontinence. Your doctor may not suggest a bladder test if your incontinence has a simple explanation, such as a urinary tract infection. In this case, you would take a course of antibiotics and be reassessed after finishing it. If, however, initial treatment has not worked or the doctor suspects the causes of your incontinence to be more complex, then a bladder test is worth considering.

A bladder test is usually performed in the doctor's office or at an outpatient surgicenter. Figure 12 illustrates a bladder test being performed. During the test, a woman remains awake so that she can describe the sensations in her bladder throughout the procedure. The information the woman provides helps her and her doctor determine whether the test reproduces her incontinence symptoms. The test should not be painful, although women with an active bladder infection or with chronic inflammation of the bladder wall (called *interstitial cystitis*) will feel some pain. In these instances, the test should not be done or should be done only with great caution by an experienced physician or nurse.

A bladder test consists of two phases, the first to evaluate bladder storage and pressure as the bladder fills (a cystometrogram) and the second to evaluate urine flow and bladder pressure as it empties (flow test, or pressure-flow test). The complete test usually takes 10–20 minutes. You may be asked to come to your appointment with a full bladder or an empty bladder, and depending on which it is, you will do either the bladder filling or bladder emptying first. Here, we describe the bladder filling first.

At your appointment, a nurse will explain the steps of the procedure, including the information you will be asked to provide during the test. Ask as many questions as you need to. You will then undress from the waist down, be provided with a gown, and be asked to sit or lie on the examining table. The nurse will first clean the area with a moist wipe and then insert a catheter (a thin, flexible tube) into the bladder by threading the tube up the urethra. This does not hurt, but it can feel uncomfortable and give you the sensation of mild pressure in the lower pelvis. The nurse may also insert another catheter into the vagina or into the rectum. Each catheter connects to a computer that collects and stores information during the test.

If you have any urine in your bladder, the nurse will drain it through the catheter before the doctor begins the filling test. To fill the bladder, a pump slowly trickles room-temperature water through the bladder catheter. Sensors on the catheter measure how much pressure builds up inside the bladder while it fills, and the catheter in the vagina or rectum measures pressure around the bladder. The doctor will want to know what you are feeling as your bladder fills. At

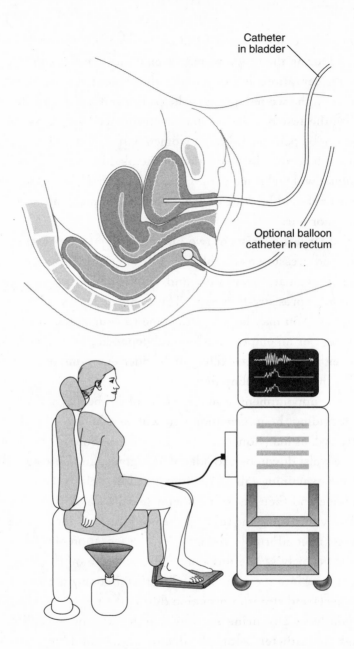

Figure 12. Urodynamic test on patient

first you may feel nothing or only a slight coolness from the water. You will be asked to report when you feel each of four stages:

1. *First sensation:* when you can first tell that water is entering your bladder.
2. *First desire to urinate:* when there is enough pressure that you would normally consider going to a toilet. For example, think about being in an unfamiliar shopping mall and you start wondering where to find the bathroom, although you don't yet need to go urgently.
3. *Strong urge to urinate:* when you really need to go to the toilet. It is akin to the feeling when you are standing in a long checkout line and suddenly have to leave the line to go to the toilet for fear of urine loss or extreme discomfort before reaching the washroom.
4. *Bladder capacity:* when your bladder is full and you have no time left to reach the toilet. Using the previous example, you probably won't make it to the washroom in time, even if you leave the checkout line immediately.

The doctor will note the volume of water in your bladder and the pressure readings from the catheters as you report each of these four stages. While your bladder fills, the doctor may also ask you to cough, strain, walk around, or wash your hands to find out how your bladder reacts to these stresses and activities.

During the filling phase of the test, the doctor may also measure the leak point pressure, which indicates the strength of the urethra. At several times during the filling, the doctor will stop the water pump and ask you to cough or strain to see whether any urine leaks out. Coughing or straining increases pressure in the abdomen surrounding the bladder and mimics the pressure that occurs when a woman exercises, lifts a heavy object, or squats down and experiences stress incontinence. A low leak point pressure means that the urethra is not strong enough to resist the abdominal pressure and allows urine to seep out. Alternatively, the doctor may perform a slightly different test to obtain this information, whereby a small catheter is pulled slowly through the urethra to measure the pressure of the urethra's walls on the catheter. This test is called a urethral pressure profile and is not as common as the leak point pressure test.

When the bladder-filling phase of the test is complete, the doctor will measure the speed and pattern of urine flow as you empty your bladder while sitting on a specially designed chair. A flow meter on the chair measures how quickly you pass the urine and how much you release. For some women, it can be extremely difficult to relax sufficiently to urinate like this, so the doctor will take your apprehension into account when interpreting the results. If the bladder-emptying phase of the test is done after the bladder filling, then the catheters are usually left in place. The pressure recorded by these catheters indicates how strongly the bladder contracts while emptying and whether you strain to assist the flow of urine. When you have finished urinating, the doctor or nurse may use the bladder catheter to drain any urine that remains in the bladder to determine whether incomplete emptying is a problem.

Finally, the doctor will often assess the support at the bladder neck, where the urethra joins the bladder, using a cotton swab moistened with anesthetic gel. The swab is inserted into the urethra about 1½ inches to measure the angle it makes with the horizontal both at rest and while bearing down.

Bladder testing most often involves only the procedures described above, but occasionally a physician will simultaneously take an X-ray or do an ultrasound. Only a few specialized centers have this capability, however.

The patient is often given an antibiotic after a bladder test, although people at low risk rarely develop an infection. People at high risk are those who have residual urine volumes, high-pressure urination, and predisposition to urinary infection. If a woman regularly receives antibiotic treatment for dental procedures because of a heart murmur, heart valve replacement, or artificial joint replacement, she should take antibiotics an hour before having a bladder test.

# Cystoscopy

Sometimes a doctor will want to look inside the bladder and urinary tract using a special instrument called a cystoscope (Figure 13). Cystoscopy examinations are usually carried out by a urologist, although some gynecologists have also received specialized training to conduct the procedure and interpret the findings. Many doctors do not perform cystoscopy examinations because they believe that the visual information is of no additional benefit when information about bladder function and urethral strength is already available from the bladder test and imaging. However, we think cystoscopic examinations have several advantages and are advisable in certain situations. First, a visual inspection of the bladder gives the physician a thorough appreciation of the appearance and quality of the patient's tissues. Second, one possible treatment — injection of bulking agents — is usually administered through a cystoscope. We describe this treatment in Chapter 6. Finally, if the patient undergoes surgical treatment and a complication arises, the surgeon is already familiar with the bladder.

A cystoscopic examination can be performed quickly and easily in an office setting using a local anesthetic (an anesthetic that numbs only a part of the body while the person remains conscious). The anesthetic is a gel administered through the urethra using a small tube like a toothpaste tube. The gel freezes the urethra and the first inch or so of the floor of the bladder near the trigone, the sensitive part. Cystoscopy is generally not painful, provided a skilled examiner uses some lubricant and a small instrument (7 or 8 millimeters in diameter).

Some doctors, ourselves included, will perform cystoscopy at the same time as the bladder test. The entire examination rarely takes longer than 30 minutes; the patient can walk in and walk out and can drive herself home afterward. However, some insurance and third-party payers will not pay for an examination of this sort unless it is done in an operating room, in which case the doctor usually administers a sedative for conscious sedation or a general anesthetic (an anesthetic that numbs the entire body and makes the person unconscious). The use of a general anesthetic increases the cost, overall lo-

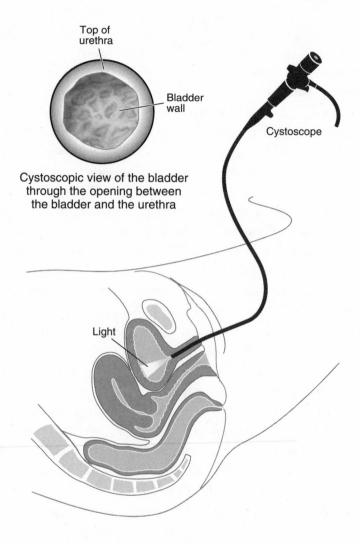

Top of
urethra

Bladder
wall

Cystoscope

Cystoscopic view of the bladder
through the opening between
the bladder and the urethra

Light

Figure 13. Cystoscopy examination

gistics, and risk (from the anesthesia) of what is otherwise a simple procedure. However, a general anesthesia may sometimes be needed for evaluation.

The cystoscope itself is made of rigid steel with a diameter of about 7 or 8 millimeters — similar to the diameter of a standard pencil. Some newer scopes are made of a flexible material. Because of the anesthetic, you should not feel any pain during the cystoscopy. It takes the doctor only a few minutes to examine the bladder. He or she will also look at the urethra while inserting or removing the cystoscope. Some water will probably escape through the urethra as the doctor performs this part of the examination.

When the cystoscopy examination is complete, you may be given an antibiotic medication to minimize the risk of infection. It is also a good idea to drink plenty of water to help wash out the bladder. You may feel some irritation in the bladder or urethra when you first urinate after the procedure, but it should subside quickly.

## Imaging

Like cystoscopy, imaging is an optional test that can be used in the evaluation of urinary incontinence. The three techniques used are X-ray, ultrasound, and MRI, all of which provide information about the appearance, shape, and position of the bladder and urethra. Most women evaluated and treated for incontinence will not undergo imaging tests, but they are useful in instances when a woman has had a poor result from treatment, when the original symptoms recur after treatment, or when a special problem exists and the physician requires anatomical information to decide on an appropriate treatment.

X-ray was the earliest imaging technique used to assess the bladder and urinary tract. Soft tissues are difficult to see on an X-ray, so a liquid containing barium (an element similar to calcium) was infused into the bladder through a catheter, and a chain of small metal beads was threaded into the urethra. The barium and metal beads showed up clearly on the X-ray. Because they were difficult to work with, the barium has been replaced with iodine and the beads with a thin plastic catheter or with nothing at all. The iodine is put into the bladder with a catheter, and after the test it is urinated out. The iodine is harmless, unless the person has an iodine allergy.

The iodine in the bladder blocks the passage of X-rays and provides a contrast on the X-ray film. However, the iodine and catheter do not show up as well on an X-ray as the barium and beads did, so the X-ray information is not as valuable as it once was in evaluating and treating incontinence. Nevertheless, X-rays remain popular because they are available everywhere and are the least expensive imaging technique.

Ultrasound is a safe alternative to X-ray for seeing detailed images of organs and other structures inside the body. The ultrasound technique uses sound waves that are sent into the body and recorded as they bounce back. Many women have their first experience with ultrasound during pregnancy, when they see images of their developing baby. In a woman who has urinary incontinence, an ultrasound shows the position and movement of the urethra and bladder. To date, ultrasounds have been used more often for research into incontinence than for evaluation and treatment of patients. We think that ultrasounds will become more widely used in the future, however, because they are noninvasive and extremely safe.

Magnetic resonance imaging uses a magnetic field to create detailed images of internal organs and other structures. The images can be taken while a woman lies or sits at rest and while she strains, so the doctor gets information about how the bladder and urinary tract look and move in different situations. As with ultrasound, few women with incontinence currently undergo MRI testing. Those who do usually have a specialized problem, such as a prolapse associated with incontinence, a failed previous repair, or the possibility of an abnormality within the pelvis. A surgeon may wish to have specialized anatomical knowledge about the pelvis before undertaking a nonroutine operation such as removal of a complex urethral diverticulum (a pouch or pocket in the urethra) or exploration to repair complications from a previous operation.

There are few known risks associated with MRI, except if a person has magnetic implants in his or her body, but this is rare because most implants (e.g., artificial joints) are nonmagnetic. An MRI offers the advantage of providing more soft-tissue detail and a larger viewing field, although an ultrasound gives an opportunity to capture movement in real time. Given the high cost, it's unlikely that MRIs will be used more frequently in the future to evaluate women with incontinence, except in specialized facilities.

*A Woman's Guide to Urinary Incontinence*

Your doctor may recommend that you undergo one or several of the tests described in this chapter. With the combined information from your medical history, the physical examination, and the results of medical tests, your doctor will be able to diagnose the cause of your incontinence and suggest possible treatments. Treatment options are described in the next chapter.

## ❧ 6 ❧

# *Nonsurgical Treatments:*
# *What Options Are Available?*

Treatment options for incontinence vary as widely as the symptoms and causes of incontinence. The options range from the noninvasive — absorbent pads and exercises to strengthen the pelvic muscles — to highly invasive surgical treatments. In between, an array of treatments includes bladder retraining, medications, products inserted into the vagina or urinary tract, and materials injected into the urethra. It's entirely feasible to start with noninvasive or minimally invasive treatments and gradually try other treatments if your incontinence worsens. Some treatments can be useful no matter what type of incontinence you have, while others are specific to a particular type. In this chapter, we discuss treatments that don't involve surgery, and Chapter 7 discusses surgical operations.

## Incontinence Products
### *Absorbent Pads*

Numerous incontinence products are available and can be useful in a variety of situations. For example, you may have only a small amount of leakage, you may be waiting for or recovering from surgery, or you may decide that you don't want to undergo an invasive procedure at present. In addition, surgery or other therapies are not always a desirable option in some cases, and the best course of action may be simply to manage the incontinence rather than try to treat it. Available products for absorbing leaks include liners, pads, padded panties, adult diapers, undergarments, and underpads (Figure 14), some of which are available in both disposable and reusable forms.

The products vary in absorbency and in capacity. Liners and pads are suited for light to moderate loss of urine and are held in place by well-fitted underwear. Some are available with an adhesive backing to prevent them from moving during increased activity and a waterproof backing for increased effectiveness. Liners usually absorb an average of about 5 milliliters (about ⅙ ounce) of fluid, while regular pads absorb 5 to 20 times this volume. Though these liners and pads sound similar to menstrual hygiene products, menstrual products are often not the best choice for dealing with incontinence because they use a different type of absorbent material and absorb less liquid. For heavier incontinence, there are also panties that come with a pocket

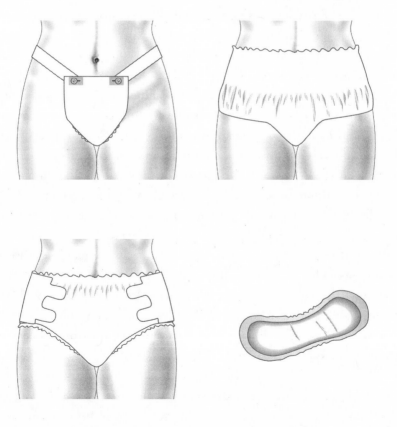

Figure 14. Typical absorbent pads and products

to insert disposable pads, which are both thicker and wider than regular incontinence pads. The panties can be laundered and fresh pads inserted.

Adult diapers are usually quite large with an outer plastic shell and self-adhesive tapes to secure them. They are a good choice for slow but significant loss of urine because they can absorb as much as 200 milliliters of liquid (nearly 7 ounces). In case of heavy and sudden loss of a large amount of urine, briefs can provide a more secure alternative — briefs have elastic around the leg, which diapers don't have. All these various undergarments come in different styles that allow them to be held independently in place by a waistband, buttons, Velcro, or snaps.

A stretch-mesh brief can be effective for holding in place any type or shape of liner, pad, or undergarment. A stretch-mesh brief looks like a fish net or wide mesh gauze of the type commonly used for surgical dressings. Underpads, which are usually used to protect bedding and furniture, are absorbent on one side and waterproof on the other side.

These incontinence products are available at drugstores and most large supermarkets, as well as through mail-order catalogs, online stores, and medical/surgical supply houses. The Resources section at the end of the book lists some organizations that compile information about incontinence products. The choice of which product to use will be a personal one, based on the degree of incontinence you have and on what feels most comfortable and secure. Many women dislike diapers and large undergarments because they are concerned about how bulky and visible these products are. Often, wearing a skirt rather than pants helps to reduce their visibility. The plastic in some products may make a sound as you walk or sit down, so this may also influence your choice of product. Cost will most likely be a factor for you to consider as well; in general, the greater the absorbency of a product, the higher the cost.

When you use incontinence products, it's critical to care properly for the skin of the perineum and vulva (the outer lips of the vagina). Urine itself will irritate the skin, and the effects of frequent moisture and drying will also cause irritation and discomfort. As well, various

*A Woman's Guide to Urinary Incontinence*

chemicals may be added to some products, including gels to increase the volume absorbed and other chemicals to reduce odor, and these may irritate the sensitive skin in the area. A number of creams and lotions are available to help protect the skin and prevent it from breaking down or becoming infected. You may find that some children's products, such as A&D Ointment, which prevents and treats diaper rash, work well for you. Although costly, changing pads, panties, or diapers frequently will minimize the risk of infection and irritation. As much as possible, keep the area clean and dry. Castile soap without irritants is an excellent cleanser to use, and it often helps to either blot gently or use a hair dryer to dry the area. Also, apply cornstarch rather than talc, which contains silicone and can irritate the skin. If a rash or redness develops, it should be seen by your doctor, who will advise you on how it should be treated.

Odor is another issue that many women are concerned about. A variety of deodorizing products, some incorporated in absorbent pads and others not, can be used to eliminate odors. Pills are also available that can be taken orally to alter the smell of urine. The pills contain a water-soluble form of plant chlorophyll. Although it's unlikely that they pose any risks, these pills are an over-the-counter product and have not been tested by the Food and Drug Administration (FDA).

### Plugs and Pessaries

In addition to products that absorb leaked urine, there are other products that can block or contain urine. These include the disposable urethral cap, urethral patch, and urethral plug. These products tend to be recommended only sporadically by physicians as temporary improvements to reduce leakage volume, and they are not usually tested using a large number of people. Generally, caps, patches, and plugs have to be changed after every urination, so many women find them too inconvenient to use after only a short period of time.

Some women with mild stress incontinence limited to certain physical activities can often gain complete urinary control by simply inserting a tampon to restrict movement of the bladder neck. A downside to using tampons is their high absorbency, which limits the length of time they can be used before causing irritation. Other devices, such as pessaries, can also be used to provide stability in the pelvic region. A pessary is a reusable, plastic insert that fits into the vagina to stabilize it and help support the uterus, bladder, or rectum. A pessary can be used to correct or at least stabilize a prolapsed organ temporarily, provided the perineum itself is strong. Although pessaries can help prolapse, they don't usually help incontinence very much. They also need to be fitted by an expert and have to be changed regularly.

Pessaries come in a variety of shapes and sizes—some are inflatable (balloon pessaries), while others are a fixed shape and size (Figure 15). You will probably need to try several until you find the one that fits and works best for you. To benefit from it, the pessary must fit well; if it falls out frequently when you exercise or lift an object, try a different one. Your health care provider will monitor you while you are using the pessary to check for improper sizing, infection, and irritation of the vaginal walls. You will also have to have it changed periodically by the doctor. A pessary cannot usually be used indefinitely because it can eventually harm the vaginal walls.

The use of inflatable balloon pessaries is limited in elderly people because their vaginal vault tends to be smaller. In some cases, a pessary can actually worsen incontinence by elevating and straightening

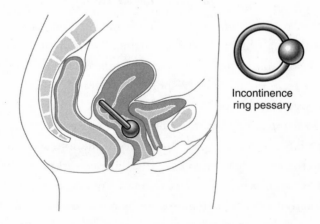

Incontinence
ring pessary

Figure 15. Incontinence ring pessary

*A Woman's Guide to Urinary Incontinence*

the urethra and exposing it to the full force of increases in abdominal pressure. However, if it occurs, this worsening of incontinence is temporary, lasting only until the pessary is removed.

*Linda was a 41-year-old woman who had made the choice not to have children. One of her greatest joys was playing tennis with her partner and with friends. She was also active in other sports, including bicycling, hiking, and sailing. She began noticing that she lost small amounts of urine when she played tennis but not when she engaged in other activities. Initially, she found that she could manage her bladder well by emptying it before a tennis game, but the leakage became progressively worse. She tried using pads but found them uncomfortable and awkward while playing tennis.*

*Linda contemplated going to her physician, but in the meantime she confided in a friend about her leakage problem. She also told her friend that she was hesitant to consult a physician because she was adamant about avoiding surgery. Her friend suggested that she try inserting a vaginal tampon while she played tennis. Linda tried this and discovered that it kept her dry throughout the entire tennis game.*

### Catheters and Clean Intermittent Self-Catheterization

A catheter is a tube used to drain urine from the bladder. The two kinds most commonly used today are the Foley catheter and the straight catheter. A third kind, the suprapubic catheter, is also used occasionally.

1. A Foley catheter is placed through the urethra into the bladder and is usually left there for long-term drainage of urine after an operation or in cases in which the bladder cannot empty. A Foley catheter must be changed about once a month.
2. A straight catheter is used for one-time emptying of the bladder and is then removed. Most often, it is used to drain the bladder once in a hospital or clinic setting or by people who rely on the technique of clean intermittent self-catheterization to empty their bladder (see below).

3. A suprapubic catheter uses a Foley or straight catheter inserted into the bladder through a puncture in the abdomen just above the pubic bone. These catheters may be used when a longer or more secure catheter is required after surgery or as a permanent method of draining the bladder when it cannot empty. A suprapubic catheter also needs to be changed about once a month.

The Foley and suprapubic catheters, also called indwelling catheters, drain urine into a collection bag, which can vary in size. Many daytime-use bags hold about 300–500 milliliters (0.6–1 pint) and are emptied every few hours. Larger bags hold up to 2,000 milliliters (about 4½ pints) and are usually worn around the house or overnight and can last for six or more hours until they are two-thirds full and need to be emptied. The smaller, daytime bags can be carried under clothing, and some attach onto the leg and are easy to conceal. The larger bags can also be carried under clothing or in a separate small bag, but it is not easy to conceal them. Bacteria may begin to form colonies in the urine of people who are catheterized with an indwelling catheter, and the catheter can also fall out and get encrusted or blocked. For this reason, indwelling catheters are changed about every four weeks.

Catheters are most frequently used for people with urinary retention or with overflow incontinence. The ideal situation is when a woman can drain her own bladder using a technique called clean intermittent self-catheterization. This technique requires being able to use your hands reasonably well, being able to find the urethral opening, and keeping an eye on the clock (or using an alarm) to keep track of when to drain the bladder. With a little practice, most women find that self-catheterization is easy, painless, and fairly quick. The catheters used for self-catheterization are made of plastic or rubber, and they are generally about 6 inches long and 6–8 millimeters in diameter. The catheters are reusable and can be used for at least a month and often longer before having to be replaced. After use, the catheter is simply washed with soap and water and stored in a clean place.

The way to perform self-catheterization, shown in Figure 16, is as follows. Start by assembling everything you need, including the

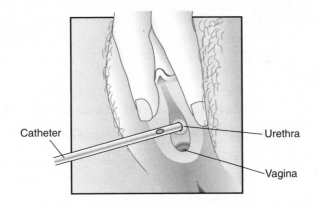

Figure 16. Clean intermittent self-catheterization

catheter and a lubricant, and washing your hands and the area around the urethral opening. Lubricate the catheter. Most women sit over a toilet as if to urinate, but you can also stand with one foot on the toilet or edge of the bathtub, depending where you are. Locate the urethral opening using a finger of your nondominant hand or using a small mirror. Then, insert the catheter gently into the urethral opening and thread it upward as if aiming for the belly button. Once about 2 inches of the catheter have been inserted, urine starts to trickle out. Wait until it stops, and then withdraw the catheter a little bit to allow any more urine to flow out. Wait again until the flow stops, and then withdraw a little more of the catheter, repeating until all the urine has been released. When you're finished, remove the catheter, wash everything, dry the outside of the catheter, and store it in a dry place, such as a resealable plastic bag.

Clean intermittent self-catheterization is a "clean" procedure but not a sterile one. Provided you wash your hands and the catheter with soap and water, store the catheter in a clean place, and in particular empty your bladder frequently, you shouldn't have problems with infection. Frequent emptying is the key to minimizing infection. Most people will be advised to go no more than four hours between catheterizations, except when sleeping. To help determine how often to empty your bladder, keep a record of how much urine you pass by using the catheter and how much by urinating. It's easy with the catheter to drain the urine into a container to measure it. (When urinating without the catheter, try using a urine hat, which is a plastic container placed in the toilet bowl to measure the amount of urine passed.)

## Behavioral Modification and Muscle Retraining
### *Strengthening the Pelvic-Floor Muscles*

The pelvic-floor muscles help support the organs and structures within the pelvis, and they are supposed to contract when a physical stress increases the pressure within the abdomen. By contracting, they help to maintain the position of organs and the pressure exerted by the urethral sphincter on the urethra, so that the person remains continent. For various reasons, discussed in Chapter 3, the pelvic-floor muscles stretch and weaken over time, making them less efficient at contracting. Exercises to strengthen the pelvic-floor muscles, also known as Kegel exercises, have been effective in people with mild stress incontinence. In several studies, people with mild stress incontinence were able to avoid surgery by strengthening these muscles. In fact, performing pelvic-floor exercises is a good practice for every woman, whether she is continent or incontinent. In particular, the exercises may be helpful before, during, and after pregnancy to maintain muscle tone and retrain muscles after delivery.

The first step in performing Kegel exercises is to identify the correct muscles. There are several ways to do this. One way is to voluntarily stop the flow while urinating. The muscles you use to stop the flow are the pelvic-floor muscles. (Stop the urine flow only to identify the muscles, not to exercise them.) Another way is to place two fingers in the vagina and contract the muscles that will squeeze your fingers. A third way is to contract the rectum, as if you are trying to hold back gas, and extend the squeeze forward. A final way is to lie on your back on the floor and raise your hips into the air, supported by your feet and with your shoulders and arms remaining on the ground. This position tightens the abdominal and thigh muscles, leaving only the pelvic-floor muscles to be exercised. Not everyone finds these techniques easy, and even after trying them, some people may not be sure that they've identified the correct muscles. In this case, and even if you think you know which muscles are the correct ones, it can be helpful to identify them through biofeedback techniques, discussed below.

Once you have identified the pelvic-floor muscles, you need to exercise them regularly — at least three times a day. There are two groups of exercises, slow contractions and fast contractions. For the slow contractions, tighten the muscles and count to five while continuing to squeeze. Then release, count to five in a relaxed position, and contract again. Keep it rhythmical. Repeat the contraction-relaxation sequence 20 times at each of the three exercise sessions. Gradually increase the time that you hold each contraction to 10 seconds. For the fast contractions, tighten and relax the muscles at least 30 times in quick succession. Repeat at each of the three exercise sessions. As you gain muscle tone and confidence with these exercises, combine the slow and fast contractions. After each slow, sustained contraction, do a series of rapid contractions. Be sure to keep your abdominal and thigh muscles relaxed while you do the exercises. Also perform the Kegel exercises in different positions — standing, sitting, lying down — to get the maximum benefit. You may find that it helps to remember to do the exercises by doing them at the same time as another activity already in your daily routine. For example, you might do them each time you brush your teeth, whenever you stop at a red traffic light, or while you are on the telephone.

If you haven't previously exercised the pelvic-floor muscles, you may notice some discomfort in the pelvic floor during the first week of exercising. Don't let this stop you from doing the exercises — keep going, and the discomfort will lessen and probably disappear with time. The more often you do the exercises, the more likely you will be to reap the benefit. Allow yourself at least three months of daily exercises before expecting to notice significant benefit, though many women notice some improvement earlier than this.

### Using Biofeedback Techniques

Biofeedback techniques are ways of learning that are used to help people retrain their bladder muscle and exercise their pelvic-floor muscles. The word *biofeedback* simply means getting information (feedback) about something biological (bio), in this case, the bladder muscle and pelvic muscles. Biofeedback training uses specialized equipment to help a woman see, hear, or feel how a particular muscle or group of muscles responds to her efforts to relax or contract them. Recall that the bladder muscle is under involuntary control — you can't decide to contract your bladder — but biofeedback helps teach a person how to have some control over the bladder's function. In the case of the pelvic-floor muscles, which are under voluntary control, biofeedback confirms that the correct muscles are being exercised, and it also monitors progress.

Biofeedback has been used successfully with people who have stress incontinence, bladder overactivity, urgency, frequency, and urine retention. For some people, biofeedback eliminates all incontinence symptoms, while in others, it greatly improves their situation. It requires time — weeks to months — to undergo biofeedback training and get positive results. Like any muscles in the body, the bladder and pelvic muscles must be exercised regularly to get and maintain the benefits.

Several different biofeedback techniques are available, as illustrated in Figure 17, including cystometric (bladder) biofeedback, pressure biofeedback, and muscle contraction biofeedback. Another technique, magnetic stimulation, uses various biofeedback signals, although it doesn't provide any feedback itself. All these techniques are conducted by a specially trained therapist, usually a physical therapist. Each of the four mentioned here are described in more detail below.

1. *Bladder-training biofeedback.* Even though the bladder is under involuntary control, there is a relationship between the smooth muscles of the bladder and the striated muscles of the pelvic floor. When the pelvic muscles contract, they suppress bladder muscle contractions. By understanding when a pelvic muscle contraction inhibits a bladder muscle contraction, a woman can use the pelvic muscles to control urge incontinence.

A therapist uses a catheter to measure bladder pressure and either an electromyographic electrode or a plug placed in the rectum to measure activity of the pelvic-floor muscle. Both instruments are con-

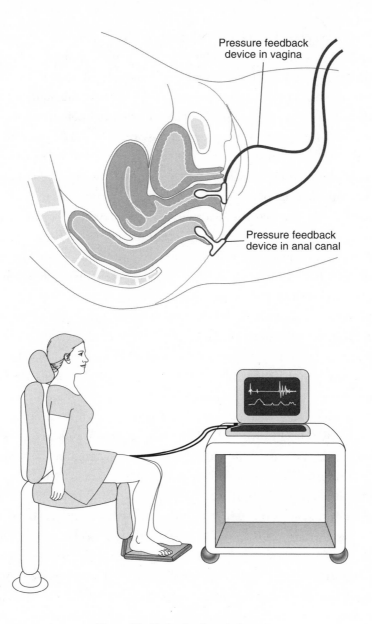

Figure 17. Biofeedback techniques

nected to a computer screen that shows a graph of muscle activity. The therapist then fills your bladder with water via a catheter to increase bladder pressure and cause the filling sensation. You can see what is happening on the computer screen as the bladder fills and the pelvic muscles contract. The graphs will show when the pelvic muscle activity causes a decrease in bladder muscle pressure. Once you can identify the voluntary muscles and the steady, persistent contraction that inhibits the bladder contractions, you continue to practice at home.

To continue the bladder training at home, you use timed urination, meaning that you urinate on a schedule — say, once every hour. If you feel an urge before the hour is up, contract the pelvic-floor muscles to try to control the urge. When you can comfortably wait for the full hour without having to use the pelvic muscle contractions, increase the interval to two hours, and eventually three hours.

With patience, time, and continued exercise, the urge incontinence can often be overcome. Initially, about 80 percent of women manage to control their urge incontinence with bladder training, but over time, the figure drops to 40–60 percent, probably because people don't persist with the exercises.

2. *Pressure biofeedback.* Several physical aids can be used for pressure feedback (Figure 18). The most common aids are plastic or metal vaginal cones, which are placed in the vagina in the same way as a tampon. The cones come in different weights, usually from 20 to 100 grams (about ¾ to 3½ ounces). The goal is to place a cone in the vagina and keep it there for at least 15 minutes while walking. To retain the cone in the vagina, the pelvic-floor muscles must contract. The benefit of the vaginal cone is that you can exercise these muscles without having to consciously identify them. This exercise should be carried out at least three times a day. Begin with the lightest weight, and when you can retain it easily for the full 15 minutes, move on to the next weight; do the same with this weight and any successive ones until you reach the heaviest weight. At this point, continue to use the heaviest weight daily to maintain the muscle tone you've gained.

Another device is a vaginal probe, sometimes called a perineometer, connected to a hand-held pressure indicator. The probe is in-

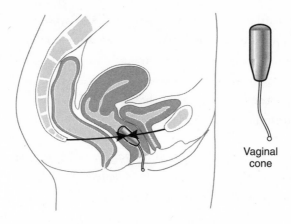

Figure 18. Vaginal cones

serted into the vagina, and as the woman consciously contracts the muscles, the probe measures the strength of the contraction.

3. *Muscle contraction biofeedback.* If you are unable to identify the pelvic-floor muscles or you can't keep a vaginal cone from falling out, your physician can fit you with a nerve stimulator. A probe goes into either the vagina or the rectum and connects to a portable, battery-operated stimulator that sends electrical pulses to the probe. The pulses are strong enough to stimulate the nerves and cause the pelvic-floor muscles to contract, but not strong enough to cause injury. You will feel either nothing at all or faint tingles as the current increases. The intensity and frequency of the electrical pulses can be altered on the portable stimulator. The electrical stimulation helps you identify the pelvic-floor muscles, and it also improves their reflexes. The stimulator can be used continuously until the pelvic-floor muscles have regained strength and then intermittently (e.g., twice a day for 15–20 minutes). Once you're familiar with the muscles, you may decide to continue exercising without using the stimulator.

4. *Magnetic stimulation.* Magnetic stimulation is another technology that attempts to build strength in the pelvic-floor muscles. Its advantage is its simplicity: you sit wearing a gown on a special chair, and it applies a magnetic current to the pelvic region that causes the pelvic muscles to contract. Because magnetic stimulation is carried out

while you sit in an unstressed situation (i.e., without straining), this technique is most effective as one component of a pelvic muscle exercise program. Magnetic stimulation is currently being tested to determine how frequently it must be done to have a benefit. It is likely to be similar to other techniques in that it is effective for some people as long as it continues to be done.

*Suzie was a 29-year-old marketing manager at a medium-sized health food company. She loved her job, was engaged to be married, and had a close circle of friends. Everything was going well in her life except for one thing: she had urgency and urge incontinence. She spent all day doing market analysis, designing marketing strategies, and attending meetings. She never had any feelings of urgency or any episodes of urge incontinence while doing these activities. Even at promotional events she had no symptoms of incontinence. The problem arose when she went home each evening. No matter how often she had relieved herself before leaving work and while on the road, she never failed to develop urgency as she headed toward her apartment door. It happened every single evening, and she was never able to get the key in the door quickly enough to open it and rush to the toilet. The worst times were when someone else was in the hallway as she returned home. She felt powerless and didn't understand how her body could betray her in this awful way. She was embarrassed and frustrated to the point of tears every time it happened.*

*Suzie used menstrual pads to absorb the urine so that she could get into her apartment without urine running down her legs. The incontinence had been happening for nearly six weeks, and so far she had managed to avoid telling her fiancé about the problem. She soon realized, though, that she couldn't go on experiencing this incontinence without telling anyone. She made an appointment with her family physician, who referred her to a urologist. The urologist evaluated Suzie and recommended that she try bladder retraining with biofeedback.*

### Using Hypnosis

Hypnotherapy has occasionally been used for women who have urge incontinence in an attempt to improve the bladder at an unconscious level as opposed to using muscle exercises and biofeedback techniques. It has also been used as a treatment to help adult bedwetters. At present, there is scant information on the use or significance of hypnotherapy as a treatment for incontinence in the adult population, but some women turn to it as a complementary and alternative medicine therapy.

## *Modifying Lifestyle*

Your doctor may recommend that you restrict your intake of fluids to help alleviate some of the symptoms of incontinence. Whether this is necessary will usually be evident from a bladder diary (described in Chapter 4). Weight reduction has been shown to reduce the number and severity of incontinence episodes.

## Medications

Medications used to treat incontinence work in many different ways to reduce symptoms related to problems with the urinary tract or to diminish the number and severity of incontinence episodes. There is no single "incontinence pill." Some medicines reduce the reflex contractions of the bladder; others tighten the sphincter muscle. Some reduce irritability or overactivity of the bladder; others reduce the amount of urine produced by the kidneys.

Today's medications for the treatment of incontinence and problems with the lower urinary tract work by affecting the way organs respond to their instructions from the brain. The nerves, which carry messages from the brain, are not linked directly to their target organ. Rather, a chemical messenger called a transmitter takes the message from the nerve ending to a receptor on the surface of the organ. The receptor is designed to accept only that transmitter — think of the receptor as a keyhole and the transmitter as a key. When the receptor accepts the transmitter, a chemical reaction takes place in the target organ to cause the desired action. A medication either mimics a transmitter or joins with receptors to block the effect of a transmitter at its receptor site.

For some people, a particular medication solves all trouble from the moment it's taken. More often, however, medication is most effective when used as part of a larger treatment program. Sometimes, for example, medication can be used in conjunction with an operation to achieve the best effect. It may take a month or more to understand how a medication is working on the body and how its effect can be used to overcome the incontinence.

A problem that can develop with medications is tolerance: the body adapts to the new medication and somehow seems to resume its old habits. When this occurs, medication may be changed or doses adjusted. Although the body may develop a tolerance to medications, the urinary tract does not become "dependent." In other words, the medications used to treat incontinence are not habit-forming, so you will not become ill with withdrawal symptoms, as with narcotics, if the medications are stopped.

In addition to their benefits, most medications have a few side effects. For this reason, take medications only under the guidance and supervision of an experienced physician and be sure that the physician explains to you the reasons for selecting the particular medication, the expected result, and the possible side effects. Some side effects may make it impossible for you to take a certain medication. Below, we discuss several medications currently available for treating incontinence, and we include information on possible side effects.

### Medications for Urgency and Urge Incontinence

When the bladder contracts at inconvenient times, it is considered unstable or, to use a more recent term, overactive. Some medications can reduce this reflex bladder activity by blocking the receptors (called muscarinic receptors) on the bladder muscle itself so they can't accept the transmitters. The purpose is to slow down and weaken the strength of the reflex response. One of the first drugs in this category was oxybutinin, known by its commercial name, Ditropan. Ditropan reduces the intensity of bladder contractions and the number and frequency of incontinence episodes caused by bladder overactivity. Ditropan is taken two or three times a day, depending on the person's tolerance of the side effects.

Side effects of Ditropan include dry mouth, blurred vision, constipation, and occasionally confusion. These side effects occur because the drug acts on all the muscarinic receptors in the body, not just those on the bladder. In addition, the drug is taken as a pill that absorbs into the blood, so each time the person takes a pill, the drug level peaks in the blood and causes the side effects. Because the drug is usually taken three times a day, the person experiences the side effects frequently. Recently, skin patches with oxybutinin have been released under the commercial name Oxytrol, and they may help to reduce the drug's side effects by eliminating the drug peaks in the blood. The patch is replaced twice weekly.

A newer drug, introduced in the 1990s, is tolterodine, or Detrol. Detrol overcomes some of Ditropan's side effects by targeting only the receptors on the bladder, not those elsewhere in the body. Detrol was shown to be as effective as Ditropan in reducing the frequency and severity of urgency and urge incontinence episodes, but with fewer side effects.

Ditropan and Detrol were both further developed into versions that can be taken less frequently but that remain as effective. Ditropan XL (extended life) is taken only once a day in a dose of 5 to 15 milligrams, and although it still doesn't have the selectivity of Detrol, its slow absorption reduces the peak blood levels of the drug and decreases side effects. Detrol LA (long acting) is also taken once a day in a dose of 4 milligrams and, like the original Detrol, acts more selectively on the bladder. Detrol LA and Ditropan XL are the medications most likely to be prescribed for urinary frequency, urgency, or urge incontinence. An individual might respond better to one medication than the other, but it is often not possible to predict which one. It is common to try one drug and then, if necessary, the other, depending on the physician's experience with each drug and the patient's particular needs.

Detrol LA and Ditropan XL are mostly used for management of urgency and urge incontinence. In carefully controlled studies, up to 60 percent of women will experience significant improvement in symptoms, with about half of these women being dry or close to dry. Usually, the improvement is described as being at least a 50 percent reduction in volume of urine lost or in episodes of leakages. These medications can be used on either a short-term basis or indefinitely.

Several other drugs are prescribed for overactive bladder — flavoxate (commercial name Urispas), propantheline (Pro-Banthine), and hyoscyamine (Levsin) — but they are not as widely used as those already mentioned. They can sometimes be useful in situations in which Detrol and Ditropan don't work. Newer and more specific drugs similar to Detrol and Ditropan, such as darifenacin, solifenacin, and trospium, continue to be investigated for their efficacy and safety. Ask your physician about these drugs and whether they are available and appropriate for the type of incontinence you have.

### *Medications for Stress Incontinence*

Urethral weakness contributes to stress incontinence and can also contribute to bladder overactivity if the urethra is too weak to contract and counteract an impending bladder contraction. Medications that increase the muscle tone and strength of the urethra include pseudoephedrine (Sudafed), a common ingredient in cold medications, and phenylpropanolamine (Ornade). They work by stimulating receptors (alpha-adrenergic receptors) on the smooth muscle of blood vessels, including those in the urethra and urethral sphincter. In response, the blood vessels and the muscles of the urethra contract and make the urethra stronger. Sudafed and Ornade have several side effects, including nervousness, anxiety, and rapid or irregular heartbeat. These side effects can be particularly disturbing to an elderly person. Because these drugs increase the risk of developing heart problems, they are rarely used and should be considered only after expert medical evaluation that includes a urologist or gynecologist.

A new drug called duloxetine recently went through testing in clinical trials. It held promise for increasing the muscular tone of the urethra by stimulating the centers within the spinal cord that are responsible for sending nerve signals to the urethra's muscles. The drug was recently released in Europe, but its submission to the FDA for approval as an incontinence medication in the United States was withdrawn because complications had occurred in the U.S. study population. Although duloxetine is approved for use in the United States to treat depression (under a different name and formulation), it is not expected to be available in the United States to treat stress incontinence for the foreseeable future.

## Medications for Combined Stress Incontinence and Bladder Overactivity

A medication called imipramine (Tofranil) is often prescribed for combinations of stress incontinence and bladder overactivity. Tofranil used to be prescribed for depression, but its side effects on the bladder even in small doses made it an attractive drug for use in children who wet the bed while asleep. The drug was found to act on both the muscarinic and alpha-adrenergic receptors, so it relaxes the bladder at the same time that it increases the tone of the urethra and urethral sphincter. In small doses (25–75 milligrams) given at night, it is an effective medical treatment for bedwetting in children. It can be used in similar doses for adult incontinence for both nighttime bedwetting and daytime incontinence, including urge, stress, and mixed incontinence. The dose used for incontinence is much smaller than the dose used to treat depression. If your doctor suggests that you try this medication for incontinence, he or she does not think you are incontinent because of depression. Rather, the small dose used for incontinence takes advantage of the side effect Tofranil had for its original purpose.

Tofranil used for incontinence has the same side effects as the medications discussed above. These side effects include overstimulation of the heart, leading to a rapid heartbeat or palpitations; mouth dryness; and confusion. These side effects can be particularly troublesome for older people. Children don't seem to have these side effects, and in healthy adults who tolerate the medication well, Tofranil can be used for years.

## Medications to Reduce Urine Production

Urine production can be suppressed by desmopressin, a synthetic form of the hormone released when the body is exposed to desert conditions. The hormone causes the body to increase the amount of water reabsorbed from the urine as it passes through the kidney. Therefore, the overall urine volume is reduced. The less urine you make, the less often the bladder fills and you experience the need to urinate.

Desmopressin can be used safely in most adults and children in tablet or nasal spray form. An occasional risk is that the body retains too much water. When a woman first starts using this medication, she needs to be monitored for several weeks to be sure that too much water isn't being retained. Desmopressin is designed to be used *only* at night and should *never* be used throughout the day because severe water intoxication can result. The medication should also not be used by people with any form of congestive heart failure, those taking diuretic medications, and those with renal or liver disease that leads to fluid accumulation.

## Injectable Bulking Agents

When a woman has stress incontinence primarily as a result of urethral weakness, injectable bulking agents are often the treatment of choice. Injectable bulking agents are exactly that: materials that are injected into the urethra to provide more bulk and resistance to the urethra's walls. When the urethra's bulk is enhanced using injectable materials, the urethra is better able to stay closed. It takes more pressure to push the urethral walls apart, thus reducing the likelihood that physically stressful activities will lead to leakage.

### *Collagen Injections*

Today's most commonly used injectable material is Contigen, the trade name for bovine collagen, which is extracted from the rawhide of cattle. Similar forms of collagen have been used for many years by dermatologists and plastic surgeons to remove wrinkle lines in the hands and face and by other surgeons as a suture (stitching) material. So before collagen was introduced for treatment of stress incontinence, the material was familiar and judged to be safe. Contigen was introduced in the United States in 1993 and has been shown to be a safe and reasonably effective form of treatment for incontinence caused by urethral weakness in women. If you are a candidate for this treatment, you must first have a skin test to be certain you are not allergic to the collagen. Extensive testing has found that 6 percent of people are allergic to collagen, with half of them manifesting the allergy immediately and the other half developing a delayed allergic reaction over one to three weeks.

Collagen injection is a straightforward procedure that may be performed in an office setting, an operating room, or a surgicenter. Collagen comes prepackaged as a soft, white paste in syringes containing 3 milliliters (⅒ ounce). It is injected through a long, thin needle with a tip about the same size as that commonly used to draw blood samples. The physician uses a cystoscope to guide the needle into the urethra and then between the inner lining (mucosa) of the urethra and its muscles. With the cystoscope, the physician can see the material being injected and continues injecting until the desired increase in urethral bulk is achieved. It may take more than one 3-milliliter syringe to achieve the desired effect (Figure 19). A liquid part of the collagen paste will be absorbed within a few days or weeks of the injection, leaving only the solid collagen in place. Therefore, the overall bulking effect will decrease during this initial absorption period, and it may be necessary to repeat the injection a second or even third time to get the desired effect.

The first collagen injection you receive can be painful, depending on the sensitivity of the urethra. The needle may hurt as it passes between the urethra's lining and muscles, and the effect of the collagen paste spreading through the tissues may hurt as well. For their first collagen injection, most women use pain medication or undergo sedation (the patient receives injectable relaxants or sedatives and continues to breathe on her own under supervision and monitoring, as opposed to general anesthetic, with which the patient is unconscious and has airway control with a mask or other equipment). In some centers, including ours, the patient receives sedative medication by injection before the procedure to minimize the discomfort without putting her to sleep and to make it possible for her to leave the clinic shortly after treatment and be driven home. We have found that a second or third collagen injection can be done with only local anesthetic jelly, as the collagen is usually injected in spaces previously filled with the same material and tends not to hurt much.

A good result from collagen can last from one to one and a half years. The material is slowly absorbed by the body and lost from the urethra, so a "booster" is eventually required. A new collagen skin test is not necessary when returning for booster injections. Just like

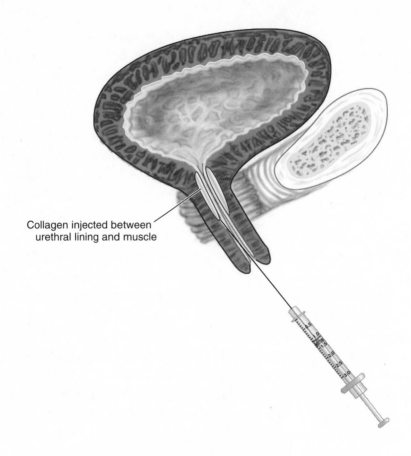

Collagen injected between
urethral lining and muscle

Figure 19. Collagen injection

second and third injections at the time of the original collagen treatment, repeat injections in subsequent years tend to hurt less and require fewer anesthetics.

As with most treatments, some complications may develop with collagen injections. The principal one is urinary retention — the urethra becomes so tightly closed that urination is not possible. Urinary retention occurs when too much collagen is injected, and it can lead either to a painful desire to urinate without the ability to do so or to an overflow of urine that produces a constant dribbling but never permits a good urine stream. However, retention is rare, and if it does occur, it is temporary, lasting usually no more than two to three days. The retention will improve as soon as the liquid part of the collagen

*A Woman's Guide to Urinary Incontinence*

paste is absorbed and the collagen is compressed in the urethral tissues. Until then, there has to be a way to drain the urine from the bladder, so every woman who undergoes collagen injection must be prepared to use a catheter for a few days after the injection. The technique is called clean intermittent self-catheterization and was described earlier in this chapter. The collagen is soft and gives way easily, so it is not difficult to thread the catheter through the urethra.

Fewer than 1 in 10 women have to use self-catheterization after collagen injection, but it's best to be prepared for it and to leave the treatment center with a catheter and an understanding of how to use it. Ask for a demonstration of how to use the catheter, written instructions, and a contact phone number so that you can reach someone in case you have difficulty using the catheter. If you have problems and go to the emergency room (which you must do if you can't contact anyone to help you), the emergency room staff may insert a catheter to be left in place. However, it is not advisable to have a catheter left in the urethra for a few days because the collagen will mold around the catheter, eliminating the effects of the injection.

There is always a possibility, however minor, of infection following a collagen injection. In our center, we usually give a one- or two-day course of oral antibiotics to cover the procedure.

Collagen injection is a relatively safe, easy, and effective form of treatment suitable for women of all ages. It may be the treatment of choice when urethral weakness is the primary cause of incontinence. It is an excellent way to treat urethral weakness in an older woman who is not well enough to go through surgery or who simply doesn't want to have an operation. Collagen injection is often an excellent choice for younger women who want to put off surgery until a more convenient time but who still want some relief from incontinence, even if it's temporary.

### Injection of Other Materials

Although collagen injections are the most common, several other materials are available, a number of them considered permanent, though none has yet found the widespread acceptance of collagen. Teflon is an older material used as a urethral bulking agent, but it was very thick at room temperature and so was difficult to inject. Teflon produced a strong reaction in the body and was later found to migrate to distant parts of the body. As a result, it never became a popular treatment.

Small silicone particles, a little bit too large to be reabsorbed by the body, have been used in France and England to add bulk to the urethra, but after the difficulties faced by manufacturers of silicone breast implants, it is uncertain whether the silicone particles will be approved for use in the United States.

A few years ago, carbon-coated latex rubber particles (Dura-Sphere) were introduced in the hope that the more permanent material would outlast collagen and reduce or eliminate the need for further treatment. Dura-Sphere was as effective as collagen, but the results did not appear to last much longer. Dura-Sphere also turned out to be more difficult to inject than the softer collagen paste, and there have been reports of the material migrating to other parts of the body, raising concerns about long-term effects. However, the material is nonallergenic and can be used in people with an allergic reaction to collagen. Given industry's interest in the treatment of stress incontinence, further improvement in this type of product is likely.

Finally, there are some advances in using materials from a person's own body for urethral bulking. These materials include ear lobe collagen (cartilage) and muscle cells from other parts of the body, but the process is still at the experimental stage.

*Charlene was 78 years old and had had two children in her late twenties. She had signs of early Alzheimer disease, but she was still quite active and could dress herself, walk without assistance, and go out with her husband and friends. Her husband, Lou, a retired physician and Charlene's primary caregiver, noticed that his wife was beginning to experience episodes of incontinence. Whenever she coughed or walked, she had some leakage. Lou bought absorbent pads and encouraged Charlene to use them; she did and went through several each day. Charlene found that when she leaked, she felt a sudden need to run to the toilet to keep from getting wet. Her doctor diagnosed urge incontinence and prescribed a medication to reduce overactive bladder. The medication didn't help much, so Lou found a specialist for Charlene.*

*A Woman's Guide to Urinary Incontinence*

The specialist did a bladder test and found that Charlene was losing the ability to feel her bladder filling. In addition, as a result of aging and childbirth, her urethra did not resist leakage as well as it used to. There were no overactive contractions of the bladder during the filling phase of her bladder test. Charlene's bladder had a good capacity, but she stored nearly 475 milliliters (1 pint) of urine in her bladder before she felt the need to urinate, and by the time her bladder volume had increased to this level, any amount of coughing or movement that raised her abdominal pressure resulted in leakage of urine. When she was specifically asked to empty her bladder, however, she could do so with good bladder pressure, and she emptied completely with no residual urine left in the bladder. The specialist diagnosed the primary cause of Charlene's leakage as urethral weakness, with the loss of bladder sensation allowing the bladder to fill too much. It was not an overactive bladder but rather an underactive bladder.

Although Charlene could have had an operation to correct her urethral weakness, both she and Lou wanted to avoid surgical treatment. Instead, Charlene's treatment consisted of small amounts of collagen injection to increase her urethral resistance along with scheduled urination, with Lou reminding her to empty her bladder at the scheduled times. Charlene and Lou also tried using an oven timer to remind her when to empty her bladder. The collagen injection was repeated 20 months after the initial injection. Through this combination of treatment methods, Charlene's leakage episodes decreased, and she needed fewer and less bulky pads during the day.

A number of the treatments and management options discussed in this chapter may take several weeks or months to show a positive effect. A woman may need to be diligent in practicing pelvic muscle exercises or in altering her lifestyle, or she may need to be patient as her physician fine-tunes her medication dose or finds the best-fitting pessary. For many women, though, it is worth persevering with the adjustments in order to avoid surgical treatment. Sometimes, however, surgery — the subject of the next chapter — is the treatment of choice for incontinence.

# 7

# Surgical Treatments:
# What Does Incontinence Surgery Involve?

So far, we have discussed forms of treatment that might be considered conservative, or at least reversible. If the use of a pessary or a particular medication, or even the injection of collagen, doesn't work, chances are you can stop the treatment and go back to the way you were. When it comes to surgery, we enter a new level: if an operation doesn't go well or produce the desired effect, it's hard to "undo" it. So before making a decision, it's important to understand what surgical operations can and can't do. In general, operations are designed to improve the function of a part of the body by changing its structure. Operations can correct incontinence in specific situations, but not all improper function can be corrected by changing the structure of the body. Most incontinence operations, including the suspension and sling operations described in detail below, treat stress incontinence, but there is one surgical option included in the discussion — implantation of an Interstim device — to treat urge incontinence.

## Categories of Incontinence Operations

More than a hundred operations are designed to repair urinary incontinence in women. Almost all of them fall into one of two categories, depending on how the urethra is supported (Figure 20):

1.  Indirect support, or suspension, operations suspend the vaginal wall without placing anything under the urethra itself. The suspension is done with sutures (stitches) that hold the structures in place much like guylines hold a tent in place.

2. Direct support, or sling, operations place a sling directly underneath the urethra to replace or reinforce a weakened vaginal wall or to compress a weak or gaping urethra. A sling can be a graft made from the person's own tissues, from biological material that comes from human or animal sources, or from a synthetic material.

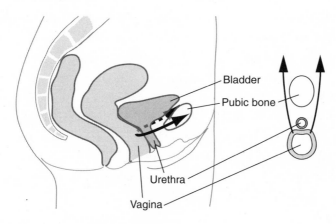

Indirect support of
urethra–bladder neck junction

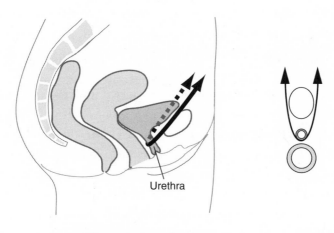

Direct support of
urethra–bladder neck junction

Figure 20. Indirect and direct support created by operations

Some operations are designed to give both indirect and direct support, including some variants of the Burch suspension, described below. As a rule, suspension operations involve less risk of changing urinary function and causing urethral obstruction than sling operations, and until recently suspensions were preferred. However, there is a growing trend for physicians to offer women with stress incontinence a sling as the primary form of treatment for stress incontinence. Slings tend to last longer and give a better result than suspensions, especially when there is intrinsic urethral weakness. The more conservative and traditional approach is to undergo a suspension operation first and then a sling operation if the suspension fails. Because good, long-lasting results can be achieved in more than 50 percent of people who undergo suspensions, and because the risk of complications from suspensions tends to be lower, a case can be made for the more traditional approach. Part of the decision about pursuing surgical treatment for incontinence involves balancing the benefits against the risks of the two kinds of operations.

## Suspension Operations for Indirect Support

There are three main types of suspension operations: Marshall-Marchetti-Krantz urethral suspension, Burch vaginal suspension, and needle bladder neck suspension. We describe the procedure, success rates, and possible complications for each of these operations below, but first we describe the general process for performing suspension operations.

Most suspension operations are performed under general or spinal anesthetic in a regular operating room by at least one surgeon — a urologist or a gynecologist — along with an assistant, who is either another physician or a physician assistant. As the patient, you are given an anesthetic while lying flat on the operating table. After the anesthetic takes effect, your legs are bent and opened. A catheter is placed into the bladder through the urethra to make it easier to identify the position of the urethra inside the pelvis. The surgeon makes a small, transverse (sideways or bikini-line) incision in the abdomen to access the vaginal wall. The abdominal incision usually doesn't cut any muscles or result in a weakened or flabby lower abdominal wall.

The surgeon then places sutures between tissues in the pelvis — the specific tissues depend on the procedure, described below. Basically, the sutures hold the vagina, urethra, or bladder neck in place by suspending them from a fixed part of the abdomen, such as the tissues around the pubic bone. The surgeon works carefully to place the sutures in strong tissues without puncturing or tearing the bladder, urethra, or vagina and to tie the sutures without too much tension. When the sutures are all in place, the incision in the skin is closed with absorbable stitches that will eventually dissolve.

Suspension operations usually take about an hour, often less if the surgeon is very experienced. Afterward, a catheter is left in the bladder to drain urine, and you go to a recovery room for a few hours until you are awake enough to be transferred to another room or, in some centers, to be discharged and sent home. Most people require at least one night in the hospital after the operation, sometimes more. The length of time the catheter is left in will vary. Sometimes it is possible to remove the catheter as soon as you are able to get out of bed, but often it is left in until the next morning.

When the catheter is removed, you may not be able to urinate on your own. This may be for any combination of the following reasons:

- The urethra and surrounding tissues are swollen from the operation. Usually, the swelling subsides within several days.
- You are using narcotics for pain relief. Narcotics interfere with the normal bladder reflex.
- You have pain and spasm in the muscles around the pelvis, making it difficult to relax and allow urine to pass. The pain and spasm usually diminish within a few days.
- You are weak after the operation and have difficulty concentrating and relaxing the muscles.
- The sutures have distorted the urethra or compressed it. Simply stated, the repair is a bit too snug, and it will usually loosen a little within a few days. (If after two or more months it remains tight enough to interfere with good urination, a second surgery may be needed to loosen the sutures.)
- Your bladder muscle is weaker than was suspected before the

operation, and it cannot generate enough force to empty the urine inside it. (For many women, normal urination takes place by simply relaxing the urethra, and the bladder doesn't need to contract forcefully. If a suspension operation increases urethral resistance too much, the bladder can't produce enough force to push the urine through the urethra.)

Most people are able to urinate within three to five days after a properly performed suspension operation. If urination is difficult or impossible for the first several days after a suspension operation, you can perform clean intermittent self-catheterization until natural urination returns. Clean intermittent self-catheterization, described in Chapter 6, is a simple technique that a nurse can teach you either before the operation or before discharge from the hospital. Alternatively, you may have a Foley catheter placed in the bladder for a few days. Leaving a catheter in the bladder for a few extra days will not make it "lazy" or weaken its ability to contract later. When there are long-term problems with obstruction of the urethra or retention of urine, further tests and sometimes surgical repair are required. We discuss additional surgery at greater length in Chapter 9, on treatment complications.

Sometimes, anesthetics or narcotics take a while to clear out of the body, and they can reduce your awareness of bladder filling. This situation can lead to overstretching of the bladder, which may damage both nerves and the bladder muscle, sometimes permanently. A woman with permanent damage to the bladder nerves and muscle may never urinate normally again, meaning that she usually has to use a catheter to urinate and occasionally may have coexisting overflow incontinence and urine retention. Overstretching of the bladder doesn't happen often, but the problem is so serious that it is worth emphasizing the possibility. Because of the potential for overstretching damage after the operation, you must be monitored to ensure that you are adequately emptying your bladder after the catheter has been removed. Sometimes a nurse will place a straight catheter back into the bladder after the first few attempts at urination to measure the amount of urine left behind. Alternatively, an ultrasound can be done to look at the bladder after urination. Simple units designed to measure residual bladder volume are also available, but they require some familiarity to use and may not always be as accurate as measuring the residual by placing a catheter in the bladder. If you are going home or to a hotel soon after the catheter is removed, you should be prepared to catheterize yourself to check on the residual volume or to drain the bladder.

*Karen is scheduled to undergo a urethral suspension procedure to correct the mobility of her urethra and bladder neck. In preparation for the operation, she had been evaluated by her family physician, who had conducted a general physical examination, some basic blood work, and a urinalysis and urine culture to document the absence of a urinary tract infection. Because Karen is of reproductive age, she also had a pregnancy test. On the night before surgery, she was advised to take an enema to clear out the lower bowel; an enema eases recovery after the operation. She was also asked to carefully wash the perineum to decrease bacteria and minimize the risk of infection (the surgeon will also apply an antiseptic before operating). Finally, as is standard practice, Karen was advised not to eat or drink anything after midnight.*

*A nurse greeted Karen at the waiting area for the operating room, and he provided her with a gown that she put on in a private cubicle. As instructed, she removed all her clothing and jewelry and gave them to the nurse, who sent them to her recovery room. The nurse asked Karen if she had any questions that her physician hadn't already answered. He then started an intravenous line in her forearm in a private, preoperative area. The intravenous line, sometimes called simply an IV, is a tube with a needle on the end that goes directly into a vein to give fluids and medications during the procedure. As they enter the vein, some of the medications cause a slight amount of irritation, but it is short lived. The nurse warned Karen of this irritation before inserting the intravenous line.*

*Next, Karen got onto a stretcher and was wheeled into the operating room, which looks like a large examining room with a few additional gadgets on the ceiling and around the room. The nurse wheeled the stretcher to a mechanized table in the middle of the room and asked Karen to carefully shift sideways from the stretcher onto the table.*

*The anesthetist then arrived and reminded Karen of the various op-*

tions of general, spinal, and epidural anesthesia. (A spinal anesthetic is a direct injection of a single dose of medication. It takes effect quickly and lasts for one and a half to seven hours depending on the medication used. With an epidural anesthetic, the medication is injected slowly until the desired level of pain relief is obtained.) Karen opted for an epidural, which can also be used for pain control after the surgery. The anesthetist asked Karen to sit on the edge of the table with her back turned toward him. She felt a sensation of coldness over her lower back as the anesthetist prepared her back and then a small stinging sensation as the needle with anesthetic was placed under her skin. Finally, she felt a sensation of pressure as the needle was placed in the space around the spinal cord to administer the anesthetic.

The surgeon inserted a catheter into Karen's bladder while she lay on her back with her legs bent and open, as for a pelvic exam. The surgeon then performed the suspension procedure, which took 50 minutes and went well. Karen gradually woke up in a recovery room, where her blood pressure, heart rate, and respiratory rate were being monitored as she regained consciousness. The nurse also checked Karen for pain, her recovery of strength, her response to commands, and her ability to move her arms and legs. Within two hours of the operation, Karen was fully awake with the pain medication keeping her comfortable.

Because Karen was to spend the night in the hospital, she was wheeled on the stretcher to her room, where she continued her recovery. She controlled her pain medication through the epidural line by pressing a button when she needed it. A safety feature prevented her from overdosing on the medication. A nurse continually checked on Karen to make sure the pain control was adequate and didn't need readjustment. The following morning, once the nurse was satisfied that Karen's condition was stable and normal, the epidural catheter was removed, and she was allowed to get out of bed and go to the bathroom with the nurse's assistance. After the surgeon had seen her and discussed a follow-up visit, Karen was discharged from hospital.

### Types of Suspension Operation

Each type of suspension operation differs slightly in how the surgeon accesses the pelvic region or places the sutures. Success rates also vary among the operations. The three operations you are most likely to hear about are described here.

### Marshall-Marchetti-Krantz Urethral Suspension

Marshall-Marchetti-Krantz (MMK) urethral suspension is also called bladder neck suspension or retropubic urethropexy. First done in the 1940s, MMK suspension addresses the problem of the bladder and urethra falling backward when a weakened vaginal wall gives way during a physical stress, such as coughing or straining. The procedure involves making a small incision in the abdomen, just above the pubic bone. The surgeon then places sutures in the tissues adjacent to the urethra and bladder neck and attaches them to the tissues lining the back wall of the pubic bone. The operation has been simplified over the years so that only one suture is placed on either side of the urethra and attached to the tissues of the pubic bone. The sutures fix the urethra in place and reduce the mobility of the bladder neck when abdominal pressure increases. Absorbable sutures were used for this procedure in the past, but today surgeons usually use a more permanent material. The patient generally feels well recovered about two weeks after the operation. The operation is illustrated in Figure 21.

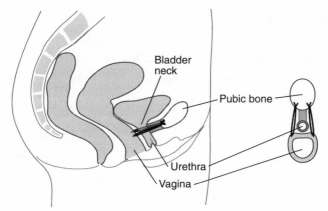

Marshall-Marchetti-Krantz (MMK) urethropexy

Figure 21. Marshall-Marchetti-Krantz urethral suspension

The overall subjective cure rates (the patient's perception of improvement, often obtained with a questionnaire) for the procedure have ranged between 70 and 100 percent. The overall objective cure rates (an independent observer finding no evidence of leakage) have been approximately 60 to 90 percent. The percentages differ because many people will feel better with improvement even though they may still have some leakage or require a pad.

Possible complications of MMK suspension include hemorrhage (excessive bleeding), tears in the bladder, and inflammation of the pubic bone. Inflammation is reported in 0.3 percent of people who undergo the operation, and it generally appears as tenderness over the pubic bone within the first six weeks following surgery. If the sutures had to be placed through the pubic bone, the risk of inflammation is higher. Inflammation may require antibiotics, anti-inflammatory medication, and occasionally additional surgery. Finally, if the sutures are placed too close to the urethra and tied too tightly, the urethra may be obstructed.

## Burch Vaginal Suspension

Burch vaginal suspension is also known as colposuspension, from the Greek word for vagina, *colpos*. In this procedure, the vaginal wall on either side of the urethra is attached by sutures to a firm ligament (Cooper's ligament) located a few inches in front and to the side of the urethra. Though similar to the MMK suspension, the Burch suspension has the advantage of not relying on the pubic bone tissues, which are sometimes flimsy and won't hold the sutures, and it reduces the risk of inflammation and infection of the pubic bone. The Burch suspension also avoids placing sutures close to the urethra, reducing the risk of blocking the urethra. With this procedure, the stabilized vagina is used to support the bladder neck and limit its mobility. As with the MMK procedure, permanent suture materials are preferred for the Burch suspension, although absorbable sutures can also be used because the resulting scar maintains the strength of the repair after the sutures are absorbed. The operation is illustrated in Figure 22.

The overall subjective success rate has been approximately 90 percent and the overall objective rate about 84 percent. The reported

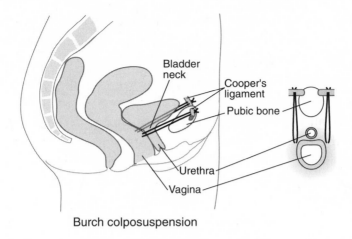

Burch colposuspension

Figure 22. Burch vaginal suspension

range is 59 to 100 percent. The Burch suspension is most effective when it is the first surgical procedure carried out (94 percent of patients achieve continence), but it still has a fairly high success rate when previous procedures have been performed (84 percent).

Complications with this procedure are similar to those with the MMK procedure and include bleeding, tears in the bladder, and the risk of bladder muscle instability and urge incontinence. Although there is a lower risk of injuring the urethra, there is a higher risk of injuring the bladder by tearing or cutting it and the ureters by causing a blockage. The Burch suspension can restore vaginal support in a large percentage of women and is often sufficient to eliminate or improve incontinence. However, the operation can fail if the urethra is very weak or if the tissues of the vaginal wall used for the repair are weak and eventually give way to further pressure or weakening over time. The main disadvantage of the operation is that it can alter the axis of the vagina and lead to the the development of conditions such as enterocele (the small bowel slipping out of position).

## Needle Bladder Neck Suspension

The needle suspension operation involves placing sutures in the vaginal tissues next to the urethra and sewing them to the back of the abdominal wall. In this procedure, a long needle is used to pass sutures up from an incision in the vagina to a small incision in the abdomen above the pubic bone. The procedure has several variants, including the Pereyra, the Raz, and the Stamey suspensions, named for the surgeons who developed them. In the Pereyra and Raz procedures, the vaginal wall is opened by making an incision and peeling away a section of the vagina to expose the urethra beneath. The Stamey procedure is similar, but in addition it uses a pledget, which is a small piece of Dacron cloth folded over to make a minipad to reinforce the vaginal tissues where the sutures are placed.

Although needle suspension operations are similar in concept to the MMK and Burch operations, the long-term results of needle suspension, for unknown reasons, are not as good. Only about 30 percent of the time do the good results last beyond five years. It may be that cutting the vaginal tissues weakens their ability to maintain good, long-lasting support. In some cases, the pledget used in the Stamey operation has been found to erode years after the surgery and has to be surgically removed. A second stress incontinence operation may then be required unless the scar from the first suspension maintains continence. Some erosions have to be repaired separately because of the damage they have caused, irrespective of the stress incontinence issues. Additional complications include possible perforation of the bladder or urethra, excessive tightness, or deformity of the urethra leading to obstruction. These operations are less likely to be offered today than 10 years ago.

## Sling Operations for Direct Support

The first operations performed on women with stress incontinence were Kelly plications (*plication* means tightening a structure by tucking in and sewing loose, redundant tissues around it). Though not a true sling operation, the Kelly plication does provide direct support to the urethra, so we describe it briefly here. The operation, done vaginally, makes a support for the urethra by grasping tissue from either side of the vagina and sewing each piece of tissue together underneath the urethra. This procedure narrows the urethra's channel and shortens the amount of vagina on which the urethra rests. Effectively, it elevates and fixes the urethra in place so that it can't move when abdominal pressure increases.

The subjective cure rates of Kelly plications have ranged between 30 and 95 percent. There have been reports of 65 percent cure rates following repeat surgery, meaning that the Kelly plication is performed for a second time. The main advantage of the Kelly plication is the low rate of complications, primarily bleeding. In addition, there is a low incidence of symptoms of overactive bladder following the procedure. Occasionally, a fistula, or passage, appears between the urethra and the vagina and has to be repaired. The main disadvantage with the Kelly plication is its poor performance in the long term, as the incontinence returns anywhere from two to five years after the operation. Nonetheless, its use is sometimes appropriate for an elderly woman, with associated vaginal surgery, or when only a minimal operation is desired.

A true sling operation places either a natural or a synthetic material directly behind or underneath the urethra to provide support and sometimes to narrow the urethra's opening. To pass the sling between the urethra and the vagina, the tissues joining these two structures must be separated by cutting. This separation of the vagina and urethra increases the risk of affecting the nerves that supply sensation to the urethra, and placement of the sling itself carries a risk of obstructing the urethra and causing urinary retention in the bladder. Partial obstruction of the urethra was considered an acceptable result 10 or 15 years ago, as long as it prevented stress incontinence. However, a sling operation that completely obstructed the urethra was not acceptable, even if the woman could empty her bladder by standing or assuming another difficult position to take tension off the sling. Today, surgeons tend to place a sling more loosely, but urethral obstruction can still be a complication of the operation because of the unpredictability of the sling's final position and the degree of scarring that will occur around the sling, as well as the bladder's strength to contract against the new outflow resistance.

The operation is usually performed with a spinal or general anesthetic, but occasionally it is done with a local anesthetic and sedatives.

The surgeon makes a vaginal incision and a small abdominal incision just above the pubic bone and passes the sling through the vaginal incision, underneath the urethra, and up to the abdominal incision (Figure 23). Some surgeons sew the sling to a structure such as the front lining of the abdominal muscles to secure it, and others leave the sling unattached to heal by scarring, in which case the scar tissue anchors the sling. Sometimes, the surgeon drills bone anchors (small screws with rings to hold sutures) into the pubic bone and sutures the sling to these. It isn't known whether these variations in the procedure improve the long-term results or simply add to the possibility of complications. The operation takes less than an hour to complete.

Following a sling operation, the bladder can be drained by either a Foley catheter in the urethra or a suprapubic catheter placed in the bladder through a puncture in the lower abdomen. Unlike with a suspension operation, if you undergo a sling placement, you are usually not ready to try urinating naturally on the day you have had the surgery or the next day. You will go home with a catheter, which may remain in place for several days to several weeks. At some point during this period, you will have your first urination trial. The bladder is either filled with fluid via a catheter or allowed to fill naturally with

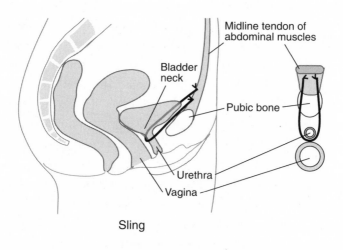

Figure 23. Sling operation

*A Woman's Guide to Urinary Incontinence*

urine. The ability to urinate should be monitored, as described for suspension surgery, once you are able to urinate. Swelling of the urethra and the effects of narcotics are less likely to interfere with normal urination in sling operations.

Sling operations have good long-term success in correcting incontinence. Depending on the selection of patients, the success rate can be as high as 90 percent. In addition, a woman has a good chance of undergoing only one sling operation in her lifetime if it's done well and it heals well.

## Sources of Tissue for Slings

Three sling materials are used today: native biological tissue (a graft from the patient), non-native biological tissue (a graft from animals or other people), and synthetic material. We describe them in order of safety, familiarity, and years of use in sling operations.

Tissue taken from the patient, called a homograft, commonly comes from the sheath of connective tissue that covers the muscles of the lower abdomen or the sheath that covers the outside of the upper thigh muscles. If the abdominal sheath is to be used, the surgeon simply extends the incision made for the sling operation to expose more of the muscle wall and removes a piece of the sheath. The piece removed is usually about 2 or 3 inches by ½ inch, and the surgeon uses sutures to make it long enough to reach the abdominal wall from the vaginal incision. A graft taken from the thigh is usually long enough to reach without the extra sutures. The sheath in the thigh is a long, wide structure — cross one knee over the other in a sitting position and you will feel it along the outside of the top leg — and a piece can be easily removed by making a small incision just above the top of the knee on the outside of the leg as part of the sling operation.

There are rarely any complications in removing tissue from the thigh; occasionally a hernia may form when an abdominal sling is taken, but this is also rare. Most often, the location used to obtain the sling depends on the surgeon's previous experience with sling operations. If the thigh is used, the operation takes about 15 minutes longer to perform, and recovery time is the same regardless of where the sling tissue comes from.

Biological tissue obtained from other people is called an allograft and from animals a xenograft. Special considerations and precautions are required in using this kind of tissue for slings, so you might wonder why a physician would suggest using any tissue other than your own. One reason is the time saved and the convenience of being able to take a product off the shelf rather than having to fashion it from a patient's own tissues. Another reason is that the product can be cut to a specific size and shape and, if small, can be prepared with sutures already in place. Doing this in advance saves time during the operation and removes some of the uncertainty about how good a patient's tissue will be for the graft.

Human tissue donated after death (cadaver graft) is the only human source of tissue (other than the patient) currently available for slings. The tissue is harvested from the muscle sheath in the same way that it would be removed from the patient. Like the cornea (clear covering of the eye), which can be transplanted without rejection from a deceased person into the eye of a living person, the muscle sheath can be grafted. However, there is concern about transmission of infectious material, including the AIDS virus and other contaminants, so these tissues are exposed to radiation to permanently destroy their genetic content and to prevent any material from reproducing once the graft has been placed into the recipient.

When a graft of the patient's muscle sheath is transplanted from one site to another in her body, new blood vessels form to supply nutrients to the graft and protect it against infection. The growth of these blood vessels increases the chances of long-term survival of the graft. Radiation prevents the development of new blood vessels between the graft and the recipient, thus reducing the chances of long-term survival of the tissue. Recent studies have also found that some genetic material can survive radiation, thus raising questions about long-term safety. While this issue may be less significant in an elderly woman, it may be very important in a younger woman.

A cadaver graft offers a surgeon the convenience of an "off-the-shelf" product, as well as slightly reducing the incisions required and shortening the surgical time. A cadaver graft rarely erodes, like a synthetic sling might. However, with poor long-term results because of decomposition of the radiated tissue, most women presented with the risks and benefits of cadaver tissue versus their own tissue would probably choose their own tissue.

Grafts from animals have been made from pig skin, sheep intestine, and cow pericardium (the covering of the heart). Grafts from all these tissues are available commercially and are approved for use as slings in the surgical treatment of stress incontinence. Here, the concern is less about transmission of infected material than about the long-term survival of the graft once it has been implanted into the recipient's body. Though long-term studies are not available to support their claims, advocates of xenografts suggest that the graft serves as temporary scaffolding — the immune system "eats up" the graft — over which a person's natural scar tissue can grow to yield a long-term repair. As with an allograft of cadaver tissue, a xenograft offers no significant advantage, other than being an easy-to-use product that requires fewer incisions and a slightly shorter surgical time.

Synthetic materials have also been used to construct slings. Synthetic slings avoid the risks and limitations of cadaver and animal tissues. The surgeon also knows the sling's size, shape, and material before the operation. For the patient, the use of a synthetic graft means less surgery done and possibly one fewer or one smaller incision.

Synthetic materials have one significant drawback: they can erode and damage natural tissues in the body. Erosion occurs when the synthetic material wears a hole through either the vaginal wall, where it can be seen or felt in the vaginal canal, or the urethra, where it permits urine to come into contact with tissues that are normally isolated from urine. Either situation can cause local infection and further damage to the tissues. Although tissue erosion is not a common complication, it can be serious. Tissue erosion usually requires removal of the sling, and it can result in further damage that requires additional surgery to correct. In rare cases, the damage is so extensive that it cannot be repaired, in which case the woman may have a catheter through the abdominal wall for the rest of her life or may have to undergo a urinary diversion (described later in this chapter).

In sum, with regard to the different sling materials available, it is generally the case that a homograft sling provides the safest alternative. Allografts and xenografts tend not to do as well as homografts. Synthetic slings, which can often provide acceptable long-term results, continue to pose the risk of serious erosion complications. Different situations may call for the use of different materials, however, so discuss the sling material and its potential risks with your doctor to determine which type would be best to use in your case.

### Tension-Free Vaginal Tape Operation

Until recently, synthetic slings were made of Dacron or Teflon, which did not stretch much and did not allow the natural tissues to grow into them well. A material that has become available more recently, tension-free vaginal tape (TVT), allows greater ingrowth of natural tissues. The operation to insert a TVT sling combines elements of the needle bladder neck suspension with the sling procedure. The use of TVT offers four new features:

1. The tape is a flexible, woven mesh of threads made from a plastic called polypropylene.
2. The tape is made with a row of barbs along its edge so that it won't move once its position has been established. The barbs anchor the tape against muscle and connective tissue and eliminate the need to sew the tape into position, giving the operation its name: tension-free vaginal tape operation.
3. The operation is performed under local anesthetic with the patient conscious. This allows the patient to cough during the procedure and the surgeon to adjust the tape to the exact location where it can produce enough resistance to urethral movement to stop leakage.
4. The tape is placed against the middle of the urethra (a little closer to the opening of the urethra than in the classic sling operation) through a vaginal incision. The tape stops the urethra's movement but has limited direct effect on the bladder neck.

The TVT operation was developed in Sweden and has been used extensively in Europe. Initial results appear promising for women with stress incontinence caused by vaginal mobility. As is the case with most new procedures, the long-term success of the operation is not yet known. In the United States, surgeons were initially slower to embrace the TVT as enthusiastically as European surgeons, perhaps because recent experience with erosion of other synthetic slings had increased their level of caution. Nonetheless, TVT and similar types of new synthetic slings are likely to increase in popularity over the coming years.

The principal risks of the TVT procedure are the use of a synthetic material and possible injury to major blood vessels in the pelvis that the surgeon cannot see when the needles are passed through. Studies to date suggest that erosion by TVT slings is far less likely to occur than by Dacron and Teflon slings, though it will take many more years before the erosion record of TVT is fully known. In an attempt to reduce the risk of bladder and urethral injury from the operation, some surgeons have tried putting the tape through the skin at the top of the leg and then threading it through a gap inside the body until it gets to the right place near the vagina. However, this method of placing the tape should be considered a new kind of operation with little information on its effectiveness and safety. Any new technique brings the possibility of unexpected risks and complications.

## Incontinence Surgery with a Laparoscope

Surgeons have attempted, and in some cases are performing, many of the operations described above using a laparoscope — a thin instrument with a video camera used to see inside an organ or the body cavity. This technique minimizes the number and size of cuts through skin and muscle. A few small punctures on the outside of the body allow access for the laparoscope and the specially designed surgical instruments attached to it. The surgeon views the camera image on a television screen and manipulates the surgical instruments while watching the results on the screen.

Laparoscopy has long been used in gynecology and general surgery to examine, repair, and remove structures that are easily visible inside the abdominal cavity, avoiding an open incision. At first, laparoscopic operations were limited to removing the gall bladder, tying the fallopian tubes, and examining the pelvis for pain or causes of infertility. In the past 10 years, however, there have been significant improvements in instruments and techniques, and a new generation of surgeons skilled in laparoscopic surgery has been expanding the possibilities. As a result, many procedures that required open operations even 10 years ago can now routinely be performed without surgical incision by using the laparoscope. The boundaries of this technique are still being explored and defined.

Surgeons have performed stress incontinence operations, such as the MMK, Burch, and sling procedures, using laparoscopic techniques. In most cases, however, when laparoscopic operations are compared with open operations, the results appear to be worse. There are several possible reasons for these poorer results. Operations for stress incontinence take place within the pelvic area, a part of the body that is not easily accessible to the laparoscope and its working tools. The pelvic organs are not in an open cavity, as are the gall bladder and ovaries; rather, they are hidden beneath layers of abdominal wall and behind the pubic bone. In addition, surgeons frequently rely on the sense of touch in performing stress incontinence operations, but they don't have this option with laparoscopic surgery. Thus, the exact placement of sutures and the strength of the tissues being sutured are harder to judge. Laparoscopic operations for stress incontinence generally require more time than open operations — additional time is needed to prepare the patient for the laparoscopic instruments and to set up the instruments and get them into the correct positions inside the patient; working within the instruments' limits also slows down the procedure. Therefore, a patient spends longer on the operating table and absorbs more anesthetic.

The advantage of the laparoscopic approach is avoiding a skin incision, but in most stress incontinence operations the skin incision is relatively small in comparison with the incisions made in operations for which the laparoscope was originally designed. What the laparoscope does not change is the amount of space manipulated internally, which sometimes may be more extensive with laparoscopy than with an open operation. The internal wound where the operation was performed must still heal after the operation.

Most laparoscopic experts working in urology and gynecology

take a cautious approach to laparoscopic repairs and select patients carefully. For example, a suitable patient for a laparoscopic procedure may be one requiring a procedure like the Burch suspension. We consider the use of laparoscopy in stress incontinence surgery to be still in the experimental stages. To date, a number of studies have failed to show significant benefits, and in some cases the results may actually be worse because of the difficulty in placing sutures without direct contact, which the surgeon has when performing an open operation.

## Surgically Implanted Devices

In addition to the operations to alter structures within the pelvic area, there are two devices that can be surgically implanted to treat incontinence. The artificial urinary sphincter treats stress incontinence, and the InterStim device treats urge incontinence.

### *Artificial Urinary Sphincter*

Since 1972, the artificial urinary sphincter, or artificial urethral sphincter, has been a widely used option throughout the world for adults — particularly men — and children who have stress incontinence because of a weak urethral sphincter muscle. It may also be used in women who have trouble emptying their bladder after any kind of incontinence surgery, such as women with a neurologic bladder dysfunction. The device consists of a small cuff, like a blood pressure cuff, which is placed around the urethra (Figure 24). A tube links the cuff to a 1-ounce reservoir of fluid placed nearby behind the abdominal muscles. The reservoir maintains a steady pressure to keep the cuff closed at all times. When abdominal pressure increases, the reservoir transmits the greater pressure to the cuff to improve resistance against leakage. A small pump on the tubing between the cuff and the reservoir allows the user to relocate the fluid from the cuff to the reservoir. The woman squeezes the pump, which is located inside the folds of tissue, or labia, outside the vagina, when she wants to urinate. She empties her bladder, and after a few minutes the fluid from the reservoir automatically refills the cuff. The device does not restrict a woman's activities.

There is a higher risk of both infection and erosion when the artifi-

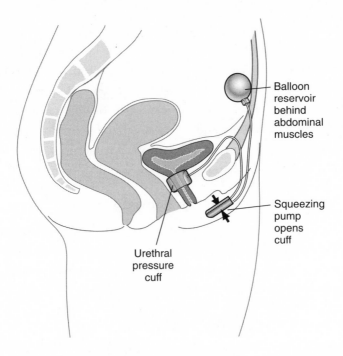

Figure 24. Artificial sphincter

Labels in figure:
- Balloon reservoir behind abdominal muscles
- Squeezing pump opens cuff
- Urethral pressure cuff

cial urinary sphincter is used in women, so it has not been widely used to treat incontinence in women. In women who have had post-menopausal changes or previous surgery, the tissues of the vaginal area have poor resistance to infection. Only a few surgeons in the United States have reported successful experiences with the device in women. Generally, the artificial urinary sphincter is not a main-stream option for women with stress incontinence, although it would be suitable for a woman with a badly damaged urethra or a high risk of urinary retention. In the case of urinary retention, however, most physicians would consider clean intermittent self-catheterization to be a safer option.

### InterStim Therapy

The InterStim device, a surgically implanted spinal nerve stimulator, uses electrical pulses to affect the function of nerves that control the voluntary sphincter muscle. Stimulating these nerves inhibits bladder contractions and reduces the sensation of urgency and episodes of urge incontinence. In a general sense, the device is similar to a pacemaker in that it produces electrical impulses to stimulate nerves. InterStim is currently approved for use in the United States for urgency and urge incontinence and must be implanted by a surgeon who has an understanding of bladder innervation and has undergone special training for implanting the device.

The procedure is usually done under local anesthesia, so if you undergo this treatment, you will be awake or mildly sedated. The surgeon inserts the wire electrodes for the device through a small incision in the lower back, activates them, and then positions them by watching the response of muscles in the legs and around the buttocks and anal area. The surgeon sews the electrodes into place and attaches a temporary stimulator unit, a little larger than a pack of cigarettes, on the outside of the body. The patient then lives with this temporary unit for several days to see whether the device works to relieve the urgency and urge incontinence. If the results are satisfactory, the surgeon implants a small, permanent stimulating unit, half the size of a deck of cards and weighing only a few ounces, under the skin above the pelvic bone in the person's back. The device runs on a battery, which may need to be changed through minor surgery after several years. If the results with the temporary unit are not satisfactory, the electrodes can be easily removed.

Initial results with InterStim therapy are encouraging, with many people enjoying a considerable reduction in urgency and urge incontinence. At this stage, we consider InterStim therapy to be a reasonable approach to consider for a woman who has urgency or urge incontinence that resists medications and is severe enough to require further treatment. As with all forms of treatment, the potential benefits of the procedure must be weighed against the risks of undergoing an invasive procedure and the consequences of living with an artificial electronic device that will likely require adjustment or maintenance during the recipient's lifetime.

## Urinary Diversion and Reconstruction in Extreme Cases

For some women, incontinence progresses to the point of being a seriously disabling problem that interferes with every aspect of life, during both day and night. In such cases, and after all other possible forms of treatment have been tried or considered, a physician may suggest an operation for urinary diversion or urinary reconstruction. Diversion operations reroute the drainage of urine, while reconstruction operations rebuild the urinary tract. These are major procedures that should be undertaken only after thorough consideration of the risks, as well as consideration of the body image and lifestyle changes they entail. Urologists and some gynecologists with special training in urology usually perform these kinds of operations.

The Bricker diversion, also known as an ileal conduit, ileal loop, or urostomy, is the most common operation today to reroute the urinary tract. The surgeon removes a 15- to 20-centimeter (6- to 8-inch) segment of the small intestine (the ileum) and uses it to form a channel, or conduit, that opens to a hole, or stoma, in the skin of the abdomen. (The small intestine is about 4¼ meters, or 14 feet, long, so removing a small section doesn't affect its function much.) The stoma is about 1¼ centimeters (½ inch) in size and is generally placed a third of the way between the navel and the part of the pelvic bone you can feel with your thumb when you put a hand on your hip. Exact placement will be a little different for each person, however. The surgeon detaches the ureters from the bladder and connects them to the other end of the newly created channel so that urine bypasses the bladder and goes directly into an external collecting bag, also called an appliance (Figure 25). The bag, which is about 10 by 15 centimeters (4 by 6 inches) and held against the body right at the stomal opening, generally needs to be emptied every two to five hours, depending on urine output.

Needless to say, having an opening on the abdominal wall and an external bag cause significant changes in body image for most people, but when incontinence is severe and other alternatives have been considered and tried, a diversion operation can bring considerable welcome relief from constant wetness. In the absence of complications, people who have had this operation enjoy 100 percent relief from symptoms of problems with the lower urinary tract, including incontinence, because the bladder is now permanently empty. The risks from abdominal surgery and possible complications with leak-

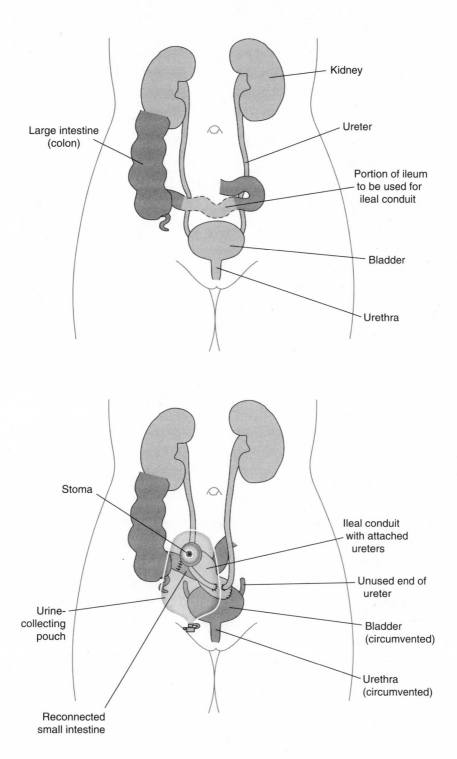

Figure 25. Bricker urinary diversion

age from the ureters or intestine are relatively small. Most diversion operations go well, but they require at least a five-day stay in the hospital and a six- to eight-week recovery. A woman can expect the diversion to last for the rest of her life, without restricting her normal activities.

Reconstruction surgery builds on the Bricker diversion but goes considerably beyond it by creating a storage reservoir inside the body to act as the collecting bag. The small intestine provides the tissue used to make the reservoir, and the opening to the abdomen (stoma) is made small and tight using a rolled tube of intestinal tissue so that it resists leakage of urine. A person who has had this surgery drains the reservoir periodically by inserting a catheter in the stoma.

Although the operation does away with the external bag, it often requires up to 2 feet of intestinal tissue for the reconstruction, as well as complex rearrangements of tissue to create a channel to the skin that does not leak. Consequently, the complication rate and the number of follow-up operations are significantly higher than for the simple Bricker diversion. In addition, a woman who chooses this operation requires considerable discipline to live with a urinary reconstruction because she must use a catheter at regular intervals. For a young woman wishing to avoid an external bag, the additional risk may be worthwhile, but for an older or more debilitated person, a reconstruction operation is usually not advisable. Even for a younger person, though, the extra risks may not be justified because most people with a urinary diversion can adapt to a relatively normal lifestyle with counseling and help from family and trained professionals.

An intermediate type of reconstruction that does not divert urine from the bladder is an enlargement or augmentation of the bladder, often called an augmentation cystoplasty. This operation is done when the bladder is too small to hold a significant volume of urine, is too stiff to expand as it fills with urine, or contracts too frequently and abruptly, leading to uncontrollable incontinence. The reconstruction enlarges the bladder by inserting a segment of small intestine into it (Figure 26). The single biggest problem with bladder augmentation is the decreased ability to empty the reconstructed bladder after surgery, since the muscle doesn't contract efficiently. The main advantage of an

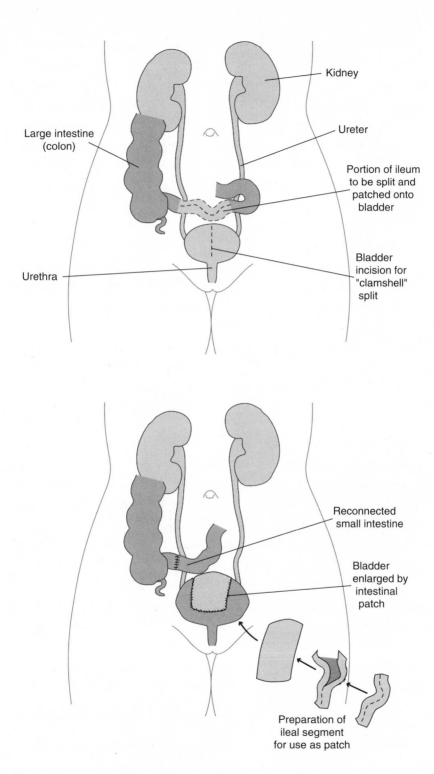

Figure 26. Augmentation cystoplasty

augmentation is that it keeps the ureters in place and avoids a diversion. With an augmentation, the person must be prepared to perform clean intermittent self-catheterization for as long as needed, including as long as the augmented bladder is the main storage receptacle for urine, which in many cases means indefinitely. Some augmentations contract later on, requiring revision, reaugmentation, or diversion. Some people also experience complications from the alterations to the intestinal tract, including changes in bowel absorption or bowel motility, usually resulting in looser, wetter stools or in constipation.

*Elaine was a 76-year-old woman who, along with her husband, was an active member of her church. She spent a lot of time helping to organize fund-raisers and social events. For about three years, she had been feeling the need to urinate more and more frequently, and this was beginning to interfere significantly with her daily activities. It got to the point where Elaine would agree to do only those church event tasks that she could do from home using the telephone. She rarely left her home, even to take a walk with her husband and their dog. By the time Elaine decided to seek help, she was feeling a strong need to urinate every 45 minutes to an hour. Whenever her bladder filled, she experienced severe lower abdominal pain that was relieved only when she emptied her bladder. She woke every hour throughout the night to empty her bladder to relieve pain. Elaine went to her family doctor, and for several months she took medication to relax her bladder muscle. She also took antibiotics to treat a presumed bladder infection. Neither treatment improved Elaine's situation.*

*When she finally saw a specialist for evaluation, Elaine's bladder capacity was 90 milliliters (3 ounces), only about a quarter of the volume the bladder should be able to hold. A cystoscopic examination showed that the bladder's appearance was normal during the first stages of filling, but after the bladder had filled to capacity, the walls cracked and bled. The specialist diagnosed interstitial cystitis, a chronic condition in which the bladder wall becomes irritated and inflamed. If she had been younger, Elaine might have elected to have an augmentation cystoplasty, an operation in which the most damaged parts of the bladder are removed and replaced by intestinal tissues. However, the operation is complicated and requires a long hospital stay. In Elaine's case, the operation would also run* the risk of the new bladder being too weak to empty, requiring Elaine to drain it herself by self-catheterization. For these reasons, and because she was older and mostly needed relief from the pain and urinary frequency, Elaine elected to undergo urinary diversion with an ileal loop.

The diversion operation took two and a half hours, and Elaine's symptoms were immediately relieved. Even though her bladder no longer collects urine, it was left in place, and Elaine has a periodic ultrasound examination (every few months for the first year or so and annually thereafter) to be sure that the kidneys drain well into the channel created with tissue from the small intestine. A nurse specialist, called an enterostomal therapist, met with Elaine and her husband both before and after the operation to discuss the diversion procedure and to teach them how to change the external collection bag, care for the opening (stoma) in the abdomen, and recognize problems.

In the eight years since her diversion operation, Elaine has had two urinary infections in the "new" urinary tract, both successfully treated with a short course of antibiotics. There have been no other complications, and Elaine continues to do well. She resumed her involvement in church activities within six weeks of the operation. Today, at age 84, Elaine is able to go out of the house when she wants to, she no longer needs to get up at night, and she has no more pain. In addition, there is no odor from the opening in the abdomen or the collection bag, and no one knows she even has the bag except her immediate family.

## Bladder Management after Surgery

As noted at various points throughout the discussion of surgical treatments, the bladder may not be able to empty itself following surgery. The length of time needed for the bladder to restore its ability to empty varies, depending on the operation performed as well as on the woman herself. Patients can expect to drain their bladder for at least the first 24 hours by a catheter placed either through the urethra (Foley catheter, as illustrated in Figure 27, or straight catheter) or through a small puncture above the pubic bone in the abdomen (suprapubic catheter). Either the patient or a nurse will measure the residual urine in the bladder after initial attempts to urinate following surgery. Residual urine should continue to be measured until the

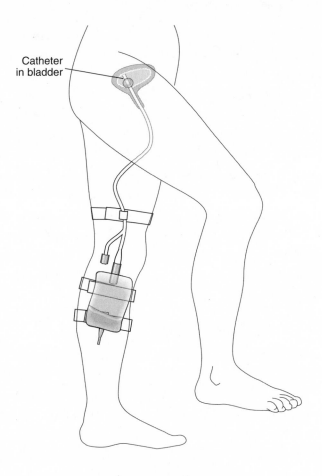

Catheter
in bladder

Figure 27. Foley catheter

bladder has recovered its full function. The bladder must continue to be emptied by catheter until the residual urine test shows that the bladder is emptying completely. Some women, like Darlene in the case study below, must use a catheter permanently after surgery.

Symptoms of urgency and urge incontinence are not unusual following surgery near the bladder. Frequently, episodes of urge incontinence result in a distressing loss of urine during the days immediately following the surgery. Medications are available to provide relief from these symptoms while healing takes place. Usually, the symptoms resolve over time.

Chapter 9 discusses in more detail the complications that can occur following incontinence surgery and when a person should seek further help.

*Darlene is a 44-year-old woman born with spina bifida, a condition in which the spine doesn't close completely around the spinal cord. Darlene's spina bifida was corrected shortly after birth, and she functioned well with rare incontinence and what she felt was normal urination. A few years after the birth of her second child, she began experiencing frequent episodes of incontinence when she jogged or did other physical activities. Her doctor referred her to a neurourologist, who found that the nerves to Darlene's bladder have several anomalies consistent with her spina bifida. The nerves don't provide adequate signals to tell Darlene that her bladder is filling up. When she empties her bladder, she does so almost entirely by abdominal straining. The urethra does not actively open and close. Instead, it remains partially open with a fixed amount of resistance that prevents complete elimination of her bladder but permits Darlene to urinate when she strains. The urethra had been able to withstand pressure in the abdomen and keep Darlene dry until, as a result of childbirth, she developed additional vaginal weakness. Though in most situations she still maintains continence, the combined effect of urethral weakness and loss of vaginal support causes incontinence when Darlene does physical activities that substantially increase her abdominal pressure.*

*A Burch procedure or similar suspension operation would not help Darlene because her urethral weakness would remain and she would soon be leaking again. Therefore she elected to have a sling, which was placed with only a small amount of tension. The operation successfully provided enough support to the vagina and urethra that Darlene was dry when she jogged. However, because the nerves to her bladder don't provide the necessary signals, Darlene has to perform clean intermittent self-catheterization. Although the nerves are no different after the sling operation than they were before, Darlene managed before without using catheterization because she'd gotten used to emptying her bladder by straining. Darlene was aware before undergoing the operation that she would have to self-catheterize, and she adapted quickly to the technique.*

The information provided in this chapter and the previous one should give you a good idea of what each available treatment involves. In the next chapter, we discuss how to select the best treatment in your situation, as well as what questions to ask your physician or specialist about suggested treatments.

# 8

## Selecting Treatment:
## Which One Is Right for You?

If you have just finished reading Chapters 6 and 7, you may be wondering how on earth to decide which treatment or management option is the best one to pursue in your situation. True, there are a lot of options, but having several options to choose from is to your advantage. The chance of finding a good treatment — or combination of treatments — is high, though as we discuss early on in this chapter, success from any treatment depends in part on your goals and expectations for recovery. We discuss a variety of issues that you should consider as you weigh your options, and we provide questions that will help you gather the most useful information for making a decision. Also included is some information to help family members and other caregivers of elderly women with incontinence. Finally, we discuss specific circumstances in making treatment decisions, such as deciding what to do about incontinence treatment if you want future pregnancies or if you also have another medical condition.

You will not have to make decisions by yourself because your doctor will provide you with information, recommendations, and answers to your questions. Ideally, it should be a decision made jointly by you and your doctor, though the final say is yours, of course. The doctor is there to discuss the options, the risks, the possible side effects or complications, and the chances of success. The doctor should be able to advise you about the different types of treatment that are suitable for you, based on your specific situation and preferences, the results of your diagnostic tests, and the doctor's experience.

The decision you make will be an individual one. One woman experiencing incontinence may decide that she wants to try only noninvasive treatments such as incontinence products and pelvic muscle exercises. Another woman may begin with noninvasive treatments and then continue to explore other options until she finds what works best for her. Yet another woman may move straight into an extensive surgical treatment. All these approaches are perfectly valid, provided each woman made her decision knowing the relevant facts about her situation and the available treatments. In addition, deciding on a particular course of action now does not mean that you can't change your mind or try a different option later on.

A word of caution: Try to avoid comparing too closely your treatment options, decisions, and outcomes with those of a friend or neighbor. Every individual has a unique incontinence situation and responds differently to various treatments. Considerations that entered into your friend's decision to proceed with surgery as opposed to other forms of therapy might have included an issue that is not applicable to you. Likewise, the suggested treatment for your neighbor might have been dictated by circumstances that you don't have. We cannot avoid comparing notes at times, but it is important to remember that no two people are the same.

*Katherine, a 47-year-old mother of three, began to notice that she leaked a little bit of urine when she exercised and when she coughed, sneezed, or laughed. She was extremely distressed by this leakage, even though it was a small amount and easily absorbed by a liner. Katherine's older sister had undergone a sling operation several years earlier to treat stress incontinence and had had an excellent result. Her sister urged Katherine to go to the same doctor and have a sling operation herself. Katherine liked the idea of a quick fix to eliminate her incontinence and made an appointment with the doctor.*

*After her evaluation, the doctor diagnosed mild stress incontinence and recommended that Katherine use Kegel exercises for several months to try strengthening the pelvic-floor muscles. Katherine was horrified at the thought and said that she wanted a sling operation to solve the incontinence once and for all. The doctor explained that her urethra was still fairly strong and the vaginal wall well supported, so Kegel exercises had a good chance of working in her situation. Furthermore, Katherine could avoid the possible complications of an operation.*

*Disgruntled, Katherine went home and thought about the doctor's suggestion. She realized she hadn't considered the possibility that other treatments were available and might solve the problem of her incontinence. After talking with her sister again, Katherine found out that her sister's incontinence had been severe with complete relaxation of the vagina and loss of support for the urethra. Katherine decided that it wasn't such a bad idea to try a less invasive treatment first, and so she began going to a therapist who used biofeedback to help her learn how to identify and exercise the pelvic-floor muscles.*

## Assessing Your Goals and Expectations

The ideal situation for any woman experiencing incontinence is most likely to return to a state of complete continence and control over the bladder. Frequently, however, this return to "normal" is not possible because the cause of incontinence is structural dysfunction. Treatment generally can't return the structure to its original status and level of function, but rather treatment compensates for the dysfunction. In addition, the cause of incontinence can often have multiple factors, so treating the leading or most likely factor may not address the others. This doesn't mean that you can't achieve dryness from the incontinence treatment you pursue, but it does mean that the treatment may not be a total cure or a forever cure. Therefore, you need to think about what a cure — or success — means for you in both the short term and the long term. If you currently have continuous leaking, would dryness under most circumstances but leaking under severe stress (such as lifting a heavy item) be acceptable? Would you consider this marked improvement to be a success?

Before selecting a treatment, especially one that's potentially non-reversible such as surgery, think carefully about what you want to achieve with the treatment. It's particularly important to discuss your goals and expectations about treatment with your doctor. He or she can help you determine what is realistic given your type and degree of incontinence. By knowing in advance what you and your doctor expect a treatment to do and how it can help your incontinence, you will have a much greater chance of success. If it helps to determine what they are, write down your goals and expectations. Try to answer these questions:

- What does success look like for me? Is it an improvement over my current situation, or is it complete dryness all the time?
- What activities do I want back in my life and which treatment can help me achieve this?
- What am I willing to modify in my lifestyle to achieve my version of success?
- What, if anything, am I willing to do next if a particular treatment doesn't provide the success I want?
- What, if anything, am I willing to do in the future if my incontinence symptoms return?

*Sarah is a 68-year-old woman who is overweight and has severe arthritis. She manages to move around slowly at home, but she uses a wheelchair to move around outside the house. Despite her reduced mobility, Sarah is an active woman who loves to bake for her grandchildren and to grow flowers in raised containers that she can easily reach from her chair. For several years, she had been complaining that she had incontinence all the time. Eventually, she became so fed up with it that she went to a doctor in search of treatment that would eliminate the incontinence.*

*Sarah was evaluated and diagnosed with overflow incontinence resulting from a poorly functioning bladder; she also had a weak urethra. The doctor suggested collagen injection to treat the weak urethra. Sarah was relieved that a treatment was available to eliminate her problem, and she immediately had the collagen injection. The collagen treatment was successful in stopping leaks, but it caused the problem of urine retention, whereby Sarah was unable to empty her bladder when she tried to. She went to the hospital, and a Foley catheter was inserted through the urethra. Sarah tried to learn how to catheterize herself so that she wouldn't need the permanent catheter, but she found it difficult to insert the catheter into her urethra because of her large abdomen and arthritic* hands. She had several sessions with a nurse who showed her how to use a mirror to see the urethra while inserting the catheter, but it still didn't work, and Sarah gave up in frustration.

After nearly a year with the Foley catheter in place, the collagen injection had worn off, and Sarah was able to empty her bladder on her own again; however, the incontinence also returned. Sarah went back to using pads, but she found it hard to manage with pads alone, and so she returned to her doctor. They discussed the possibility of a sling operation to treat the weak urethra, but this procedure would require Sarah to perform self-catheterization for the rest of her life, or as long as the sling was effective at holding the urethra. Given her previous experience with trying to learn self-catheterization, Sarah knew it wasn't a possibility for her. So, she reevaluated her options and settled on a permanent Foley catheter. With the catheter in place, Sarah remained dry as long as she was seated or lying down, but she leaked whenever she stood up because the urethra was so weak that urine trickled along the edges of the catheter. Sarah continued to use pads whenever she was standing and moving about in her home. Because she used her wheelchair whenever she left her home, she didn't need to worry about incontinence in public.

Although Sarah's ultimate treatment was not what she had initially expected or wanted, she successfully adjusted her recovery goals and found an acceptable way to manage her incontinence.

## Issues to Consider when Selecting Treatment

As we discussed in Chapter 4, make sure that you feel comfortable speaking with your doctor. If your questions are not being answered to your satisfaction or if you feel your concerns are being dismissed, don't be afraid to seek another opinion or switch to a different doctor altogether. Likewise, a complete evaluation of bladder function provides information needed to select an appropriate treatment, so if you think the doctor has taken any shortcuts in assessing your condition, consider consulting another physician before moving ahead with treatment decisions. When you feel comfortable with your doctor and medical assessment, and once you know what you want to achieve from treatment, you can begin assessing the options to determine which ones might bring you success. Recall from Chapters 6 and 7 that there are five broad categories of treatment, though the first is a management option more than a treatment:

1. Incontinence products
2. Behavioral modification and muscle retraining
3. Medications
4. Injectable bulking agents
5. Surgery

Your doctor should help you narrow down the categories, as well as the options within each category, because some may not be appropriate for your type of incontinence. If your doctor recommends only one type of treatment, particularly if it is an invasive and irreversible one, ask about alternatives. Ideally, you will be presented with a number of treatment options, and your doctor will go through them with you to discuss how each might help in your situation.

Before discussing specific questions to ask about treatment options, it's worth mentioning that a possible course of action may be no action, at least not to start with. If incontinence is minimal and not badly disruptive to your life, then management of the situation with products such as absorbent pads may be sufficient "treatment." Your incontinence may or may not worsen over time, so it could remain manageable, or it could develop to a stage at which the use of incontinence products provides insufficient relief. It's impossible to predict with certainty whether a woman's incontinence will become worse over time, but lifestyle and activities do play a role, especially in stress incontinence. A woman with a fairly sedentary lifestyle may not experience a progression, while a physically active woman probably will. The speed that incontinence worsens for an active woman will have to do with how strenuous her activities are and the amount of strain to which the pelvic organs and pelvic floor are subjected.

If you want to go further than managing your incontinence with products, there are several factors to consider for each possible treatment.

- **Is this treatment appropriate for the type and severity of incontinence that I have?**

  Some treatments are designed for a specific type of incontinence, while others can be used with several types. For example, bladder retraining will not help mild stress incontinence due to a weakened sphincter muscle, but collagen injections probably will. If your stress incontinence is severe, collagen injections may be insufficient to provide the necessary closure of the urethra, whereas sling surgery may provide a greater chance of success. In contrast to these two examples, medications are a form of treatment that can be used for both stress and urge incontinence.

- **What are the benefits of this treatment?**

  If there weren't any benefits to a particular treatment, then it wouldn't even be an option. However, some treatments are more likely than others to provide benefits, depending on the person's situation. Muscle contraction biofeedback may work well for a woman with mild stress incontinence who is able to spend several months strengthening the pelvic muscles, while suspension surgery may have greater benefits for a woman with severe stress incontinence resulting from vaginal prolapse.

- **What are the risks and possible complications of this treatment?**

  Most treatments include risk, though for some the risks are minor and for others they are more severe. The risk of trying pelvic muscle exercises is that you may not identify the correct muscles and therefore will not benefit. Conversely, the risk of some surgeries is that you may develop problems with urgency following the procedure, and some medications have serious side effects such as increased heart rate. In many cases and often regardless of the type of treatment, there are risks that incontinence will reoccur and further treatment will be necessary.

- **How do the benefits compare with the risks in the short term and long term?**

  The best treatment is one that provides maximum benefit and minimum risk, but it can be difficult to weigh the two. Sometimes, a particular treatment may have greater benefit or be more successful than other treatments, but it also requires a longer recovery time or has a higher likelihood of complications. The decision may come down to what is possible in a woman's life at that point — if she is busy caring for other family members or pursuing a career, she may decide to try a treatment that will provide relief only in the short term but that allows her to continue her life without the disruption of extensive recovery. Ideally, a person will have the time to compare the benefits and risks of different treatment alternatives without feeling pressure to make a decision.

- **Will this treatment cure my original incontinence but leave me with another problem?**

  Most procedures carry the risk of causing some obstruction, even if mild, so the benefit of correcting the incontinence may come at the cost of being unable to urinate naturally. In these circumstances, a woman no longer has difficulty retaining urine in the bladder, but instead she finds it difficult to empty her bladder. The full bladder can then lead, at times, to problems with urgency and urge incontinence. These problems can be alleviated with medications, but this may not be the outcome you envision from the initial treatment.

- **Will this treatment require me to change my daily routine or activities?**

  Sometimes, a treatment requires lifestyle adjustment or trade-offs. For example, a woman may find that an operation allows her to maintain dryness but that she has to perform clean intermittent self-catheterization to ensure that her bladder empties completely. In another instance, a woman who has undergone a diversion operation will have to come to terms with having a hole in the abdominal wall and with periodically emptying her urine collection bag.

- **What are the chances that my incontinence will persist despite this treatment?**

  The success rates are rarely 100 percent, so with any treatment there is a chance that incontinence will continue. The incontinence may be the same as before treatment, or it may be improved but still not sufficiently improved to be deemed successful. Success rates vary among treatments and should be evaluated carefully. Ask the doctor who will be performing the operation what the chances of success are for improvement or cure of your incontinence, as well as what changes may be necessary in your urination habits. Also ask the doctor to compare his or her own experience with results published in the literature and with the experience of experts. This will help you get a realistic assessment of your chances for success in the hands of the person who is treating you.

- **Where is the best place to have the treatment done?**

  Incontinence treatments are offered both at centers that specialize in treating incontinence and at a variety of clinics and hospitals that deal with many different conditions and diseases. Doctors at specialized centers benefit from seeing more patients with incontinence, and therefore they often have more experience with specific procedures. Specialized centers also tend to have state-of-the-art facilities and equipment. For most people, the drawback is the location of a specialized center, since there are fewer of them and invariably they are not close to home. The location also has ramifications for follow-up care after a treatment has been completed, particularly if the treatment involved surgery. Usually, a woman can receive excellent care by staying close to home and seeing a doctor with interest in her particular problem. Of course, it never hurts to ask your doctor about specialized centers and the possibility of being referred to one.

For many women, the decision about which treatment to pursue is not a clear-cut choice because the outcome is often probable rather than certain. You usually have to make some compromise in selecting a treatment, especially if the cause of your incontinence is complex or if it is particularly severe. You may also want to consider how many times you will undergo treatment should the first attempt not work, or how many and which treatments you will try before you move on to another option. Having treated many people with incontinence during our years of medical practice, we advise a conservative approach that begins with a reversible treatment, such as biofeedback or medication, as a first step. If the reversible treatment does not work, it is always possible to progress to more aggressive treatments, such as an irreversible surgical treatment. Usually, the first surgical procedure has the best chance of achieving good results. Unfortunately, the more surgeries you undergo, the more difficult it becomes to correct the problem. Because the decision to undergo surgery is a significant one, we next cover some points to consider and relevant questions specifically about incontinence operations.

*Cathy, a 42-year-old nurse and single mother, had had two vaginal deliveries in her late twenties. By her mid-thirties, she had developed some stress incontinence that she managed with pads. Over time, however, the incontinence worsened, so Cathy went for an evaluation. Her doctor found that her urethra was weak. Given the daily physical activity with her job, the doctor recommended a sling operation. Cathy was wary of undergoing an operation because she was so busy looking after her two teenage daughters and she didn't want to deal with the recovery period after an operation. She asked about alternatives, and the doctor suggested that collagen injections might provide sufficient bulk to the urethra to relieve her incontinence. Cathy had collagen injected, and it worked for 10 months. She then returned to her doctor for more collagen. Cathy ended up having collagen injected five times during three years, with the respite from incontinence lasting for a shorter period each time.*

*Eventually, however, the doctor advised Cathy that further collagen injections were not going to correct the incontinence, so Cathy finally decided to undergo a sling procedure. By this time, one of her daughters had left home for college, and her second daughter was in her final year of high school. Cathy had the sling operation, which was successful at treating the stress incontinence, but she developed urgency after the surgery. She had known urgency was a possible complication, and she readily tried the skin patch medication that her doctor prescribed. The medication reduced her urgency and didn't cause any side effects. Cathy was happy with the combination of treatments she had ultimately used to address her incontinence.*

# Opting for Surgery

As we've mentioned before, surgery to treat incontinence is generally an irreversible procedure. Most other treatments can be discontinued if they don't produce the desired results or if they cause unwanted side effects, but not so with surgery. Therefore, if you decide to proceed with an incontinence operation, it is advisable to consider a few more issues and ask a few more questions.

When you are choosing a surgeon, ask about his or her experience with the particular operation you plan to undergo as well as success rates and complication rates. Pay attention to how the surgeon responds to your questions and evaluates your problem. Find out about postoperative care and how much access you will have to the surgeon. It's helpful to ask these types of questions not only for the information you get but also to get a sense of the surgeon's communication ability, which can become important for ongoing dialogue after surgery.

In all states, you must give your consent to undergo any operation or invasive kind of treatment. You must be adequately informed about the reasons for the operation, the risks involved, and the available alternatives, and you must then sign a consent form indicating that you have been made aware of these points. This process is called obtaining informed consent, and its purpose is to provide you, as the patient, with protection against bad or unexpected results from operations that were entered into without full understanding of the potential consequences. To be certain that you truly have understood all the issues surrounding a particular operation, take your time to ask questions and don't feel rushed into making a decision or into signing a consent form. The questions below should help you obtain the necessary information. Because there are so many questions, it can be helpful to use a mnemonic — CURE — to remember the type of questions to ask. Here, we first list some general questions and then the CURE questions.

## *General Questions*

- What kind of operation has been proposed and what is the name of it?

- What are the reasons for doing this operation?
- What is the operation designed to do?
- What are the success rates with the operation? For how long has the operation been done?
- What are the alternative treatments?
- Is any synthetic material going to be used in the operation? Is there an alternative?
- Is any cadaver or animal tissue going to be used in the operation? What are the alternatives?
- How long should the operation take?
- How long is the hospital stay?

### C *for Complications and Catheters*

- What are the possible complications after the operation? What is the likelihood that they will occur? What symptoms should I look for to recognize complications?
- How will I manage urine output after surgery? If with a catheter, what kind and for how long?

### U *for Urine and Urge*

- What effects could the operation have on bladder function? On the pelvic floor? On bowel function?
- How long should it take to have normal bladder function?
- What is the likelihood of urgency and urge incontinence developing after the operation? Would they be temporary or require additional treatment such as medication?

### R *for Risk, Recovery, and Recurrence*

- What are the risks during the operation? What is the likelihood that they will occur?
- What is the risk of urinary tract infections after the operation?
- How long is recovery likely to take? When will I be able to resume physical activities without jeopardizing the success of the operation?
- What is the long-term outcome of the operation? How will time and aging affect the outcome?

*A Woman's Guide to Urinary Incontinence*

- What are the risks that my incontinence will recur and would the recurrence be worse than the original problem? If it recurs, will I need another surgical procedure?

### E *for Exercise and Experience*

- What type of exercise will I be able to do after the operation and still remain dry?
- How familiar is the surgeon with the operation and with treating its complications?

The case study of Arlene, below, provides an extreme example of what can happen if all the features of a person's situation are not considered before treatment. Unfortunately, incomplete knowledge in the selection of treatment can lead to unwanted and unexpected results.

*Arlene was a 58-year-old woman who had mild urinary urgency that developed over a period of three years into severe urgency and urge incontinence. Initially, Arlene had been able to cope with the sensation of urgency, but as it worsened, it interfered substantially with her job on the front reception desk of a large firm of financial investment advisers. It was both awkward and embarrassing to be continually running from the front desk to the washroom, only to return to her chair and within minutes rush off again.*

*Arlene went to her doctor, who diagnosed an unstable bladder that developed spasms when it had filled to only around 100 milliliters (about 3 ounces). She tried medications to decrease the activity of the bladder muscle, without success. Desperate for a resolution, she elected to have her bladder enlarged with a piece of her bowel. After surgery, her enlarged bladder increased her capacity to approximately 220 milliliters (7 ounces), and her urgency was significantly reduced.*

*The use of part of her large bowel, however, reduced the absorption of water from the feces before they went to the rectum. The increased water content caused extra stress on the bowel and rectum to the point that Arlene now felt the urge for more frequent bowel movements, sometimes with diarrhea. She also experienced occasional fecal incontinence. Although her urinary incontinence was significantly improved, Arlene now had a new and difficult problem to deal with. An evaluation of her rectal function showed that her bowel and rectum had a problem with overactivity, similar to what she had originally experienced with her bladder.*

*Arlene's original urgency and urge incontinence would likely have been successfully treated with an InterStim device, but this option was not yet available. If it had been, Arlene could have avoided the intestinal complication.*

## Caring for an Elderly Woman with Incontinence

Incontinence may be the reason for as many as 50 percent of nursing home admissions, in part because of the difficulty family members and caregivers have with managing an elderly person with incontinence at home. People who are very elderly require special considerations when evaluating and treating incontinence. Elderly people have less tolerance for complications of treatment, especially surgical treatment, and are generally more sensitive to medication. They are more likely to be taking sleep medications and antidepressants. They may also have coexisting illnesses such as hypertension, diabetes, and heart disease, with some medications for these conditions — such as diuretics (fluid pills), sedatives, or tranquilizers — increasing problems with incontinence. A number of medications can also cause confusion for elderly people, and this interferes with their ability to control and respond to bladder events. If a person has dementia, or simply reduced mental awareness of her body functions and surroundings, she can lose awareness of the bladder, with resulting overflow incontinence or bladder overactivity. Depending on her level of awareness, an elderly woman may or may not feel sudden urgency. She may simply be wet all the time and be unaware of it, with severe skin irritation, or dermatitis, developing as a result.

In addition to medication and other treatments that a physician can provide, elderly women and their families usually require adjustments in lifestyle. For example, they must often incorporate escorted, timed urination into their daily routines because the sensation and need to urinate diminish sooner than the ability to empty on command. Diapers should be changed whenever they become wet to avoid the skin breaking down. It is particularly important to inspect the skin periodically.

If an incontinence treatment is being considered, keep in mind that conservative treatments are the safest for an elderly woman. Collagen injection is often a reasonable option, but because most elderly women have a weak urethral sphincter and some degree of bladder dysfunction, obstructing operations such as slings should be approached with great caution. Family members must also consider who will be available to help an elderly woman after undergoing a surgical treatment. For example, a woman who is independent before treatment might lose her independence if the operation isn't successful or causes other problems.

*Mary, an 89-year-old widow who lived in a studio apartment in her daughter and son-in-law's house, had had mild stress incontinence for many years. In her seventies, she had been treated with medication and biofeedback to help identify and strengthen the pelvic muscles. For several years, Mary had been good about doing her pelvic-floor exercises. Once she got to know which muscles to contract and how to contract them, she continued on her own. She also used vaginal cones to help her with these exercises. However, as she got older, Mary often forgot to do the exercises, and when she did remember and tried to use the vaginal cones, they invariably fell out. The medication had continued to have some benefit, but as she aged, she experienced more alarming side effects, notably an irregular heartbeat. At 82, she moved into the studio in her daughter Rachel's home. At that time, Mary had stopped taking the medication, and both her doctor and Rachel encouraged her to try collagen injections. Mary steadfastly refused. She was still mobile and self-sufficient, and she used padded underwear to manage her incontinence.*

*By age 89, Mary began to experience reduced bladder awareness and overflow incontinence. She was also beginning to have dementia. Mary now used adult diapers to contain the urine, but she frequently wasn't aware that she had wet herself and didn't change the diapers. Rachel started reminding her to change the diaper, but doing so soon became too much for Mary. Rachel then got into the habit of changing her mother's diaper for her. Conveniently, Rachel worked as a freelance Web site de-*

*signer from her home and was able to keep an eye on her mother during the day. Mary was initially quite willing to let Rachel change the diapers, but she later started to fight Rachel's efforts. Because it was difficult to change her, Mary spent longer periods in a wet diaper and developed severe skin irritation. Rachel got some ointment recommended by her local pharmacist, and this helped ease the rash.*

*Rachel persevered for several months, but changing Mary was so difficult that Rachel eventually took her mother to see a doctor. Rachel asked the doctor if there were any other options or if she should think about moving Mary into a care home. The doctor suggested inserting an indwelling catheter that could be emptied to a collection bag and more easily changed. They tried this option and found that it worked well for both Mary and Rachel.*

## Specific Circumstances in Deciding on Treatment
### *Wanting Future Pregnancy*

It is often a good idea to avoid having surgery for stress urinary incontinence before completing childbearing. Sometimes, however, the incontinence is particularly distressing, and the more conservative treatments are ineffective, so the possibility of surgery needs to be entertained. If you are in this situation and decide to proceed with an incontinence operation, you should make note for when you become pregnant to discuss the risks and benefits of a vaginal versus a cesarean section delivery with both your obstetrician and the surgeon who performed the incontinence repair.

If you experience urinary incontinence that worsens during the course of a pregnancy, you may be tempted to ask your doctor to perform surgery to correct the incontinence at the time of a planned cesarean delivery. We advise against this, however, because incontinence symptoms will subside with time after a delivery, and the pelvic-floor changes related to pregnancy require anywhere from three to six months to settle down before a suspension or sling operation can be done with predictable results. Furthermore, increased blood flow and changes to tissues that occur during pregnancy can complicate both the incontinence surgery and the chance of success.

## Considering a Simultaneous Hysterectomy

When a woman has completed her childbearing and the uterus shows signs of either relaxation or abnormalities, the uterus can be removed in an operation known as a hysterectomy. If the woman also requires an incontinence operation, the preference is to remove the uterus at the same time as performing the incontinence surgery.

If, however, the uterus shows no signs of weakening support within the pelvis and has no abnormalities that indicate it should be removed, it should be left in place during incontinence surgery. There is no evidence that a hysterectomy improves the outcome of incontinence surgery when the incontinence is caused solely by poor urethral support. Therefore, it is unnecessary to perform a hysterectomy at the same time as incontinence surgery simply to improve the results of the surgery. In fact, detaching the uterus during a hysterectomy carries the risk of damaging the nerves that supply the bladder, with the possible result of altered bladder function such as urgency. So, without a specific reason to remove the uterus, it is best left alone.

## Correcting Pelvic Organ Prolapse

As discussed in Chapter 3, any one of the organs in the pelvic area can move out of its normal position — called prolapse — and may affect bladder function. If you experience prolapse of a pelvic organ, your doctor will conduct a careful examination to determine the influence of the prolapse, as well as the influence of correcting the prolapse, on bladder function. The prolapsed organ may mask other symptoms of incontinence that become apparent once the prolapse has been corrected. Correcting weakened support of the pelvic organs often requires the skills of a variety of specialists, including urologists, gynecologists, colorectal surgeons, and plastic surgeons.

## Understanding the Limitations from Other Conditions

Other medical conditions or situations often need to be taken into consideration when selecting a treatment for urinary incontinence. If you have a solitary kidney, a neurological condition, or a long-term illness, tell your doctor about it, since these conditions will most likely affect the options for incontinence treatment. Similarly, if you have had radiation therapy in the past, tell your doctor. Radiation therapy, for example, interferes with healing from surgery and pre-disposes a person to increased risk of complications in surgeries performed after the radiation. Radiation can play a role in the development of incontinence by irritating tissues in the urinary tract, and these symptoms are usually not correctable by surgery. Radiation can cause scarring through damage to blood vessels that supply muscles and connective tissues. As a result, the bladder can become stiffer, the urethra less supple and less able to stay closed, and the nerves damaged and irritable. Common symptoms include reduced filling volume, increased urgency and frequency, and occasional bleeding. The key is to bring the past radiation therapy — or other condition — to your doctor's attention and to discuss the possible implications for your incontinence treatment.

*Linda, a 37-year-old sales associate in a clothing boutique, had recurrent urinary tract infections and began having difficulty with completely emptying her bladder. She also experienced occasional leakage of urine when she picked something up, including her toddler. Each time she went to see her doctor, he prescribed antibiotics to address the urinary tract infection and suggested that the bladder emptying would return to normal when the infection had gone. The doctor also said the leakage Linda experienced was normal, given that she'd had a child. Linda's bladder emptying became progressively worse, and she felt certain that the antibiotics were doing nothing to address the problem. The urine leakage didn't get any worse, but it continued to cause frustration and embarrassment. Her discomfort and frequent trips to the toilet in attempts to empty her bladder also interfered significantly with her job and with the rest of her life.*

*Linda was reluctant to return to the same doctor, so on her husband's urging, she decided to seek a second opinion. She went to a urologist recommended by her mother. The urologist evaluated Linda and determined that the leakage was due to a weak bladder neck and could be treated with a bladder neck suspension. He couldn't find a cause for the incomplete emptying but noted that Linda also experienced some numbness and tingling sensations in her hands and feet. Suspecting a problem with nerve signals, the urologist referred Linda to a neurologist, who conducted some further tests and diagnosed multiple sclerosis. The multiple sclerosis was responsible for the bladder's inability to generate a contraction strong enough to empty completely.*

*Linda was taught how to perform clean intermittent self-catheterization, and with practice she became adept at draining her bladder quickly and painlessly.*

## Participating in a Research Trial

Before ending this chapter on selecting the best treatment for your situation, we will briefly discuss the possibility of participating in a research trial. New drugs, devices, and other treatments are constantly being developed by investigators in universities, other research institutions, and medical industries such as pharmaceutical and medical device companies. To determine whether they are beneficial, these new developments go through many phases of testing, including testing on groups of people. Your doctor may suggest that you join a research trial for your treatment. Should you participate in a research study? It may be appealing to do so, especially because the treatment is usually offered free of charge and typically includes extensive medical evaluation and testing, also at no charge. A participant often feels that she is receiving the latest and newest treatment.

In the United States, the federal government carefully regulates the phases of testing, so by the time a new treatment is used in a trial, it has already been well scrutinized. Participants' safety during research trials has become a major concern of the medical profession and the federal government, as well as of the people who conduct the trials within research institutions and the medical industry. There has probably never been a safer time to become a participant in a research study.

Some research trials are established to determine which of several treatments works best. On the one hand, if you participate in a study like this, you are an experimental subject. But on the other hand, you may receive the same kind of treatment you otherwise would have, and the treatment will be provided under carefully controlled circumstances. Your protection and safety and the results of your outcome will be monitored. So why not participate? As with any treatment decision, you need to find out as much as you can about the research study and treatment before making a decision to enroll in the study. Has it been designed for women with your type of incontinence? What are the potential risks and benefits? How long will the study last? What are you obliged to do in terms of being tested, evaluated, and followed up? Your approach to research studies should be guided by the principles outlined in this book. As in all aspects of medical treatment, you will do best if you have a reasonably good idea of what is wrong with you and if you understand the possible outcomes of your treatment choices.

# ❧ 9 ❧

## *Treatment Complications:*
## *What to Do if Something Goes Wrong*

Even after careful examination of the problem and thorough research into treatment options, the unfortunate reality is that sometimes treatment does not go as expected. The treatment may not fix the problem, or it may create a new one. Sometimes a new problem is worse than the original one. Sometimes it can be fixed; other times it can't. When the selected treatment is reversible — use of medications, urethral patches, or even injectable agents, as examples — a poor result can be dealt with fairly easily. The woman and her doctor stop the ineffective treatment, reassess the situation, and examine the remaining options. When the treatment is not reversible, however, which is generally the case with incontinence operations, the picture becomes a little less clear. This chapter is devoted to discussing the complications and problems that women may experience following surgery to treat their incontinence.

## Urine Retention in the Bladder

Urine retention means that the bladder cannot empty itself and the urine remains trapped. Most operations for stress urinary incontinence run the risk of producing temporary or, less frequently, permanent urinary retention. When the operation creates too tight an obstruction around or underneath the urethra, the urine simply can't get through. With temporary obstruction, a woman has difficulty urinating or cannot urinate at all. Her urine flow may be interrupted, she may have to strain to urinate, or she may feel bladder fullness and the need to urinate but nothing will come out. The obstruction can be due to any one of several factors associated with surgery: tissue swelling, bladder weakness, pain or spasm in the pelvis making it difficult to relax the necessary muscles, or lingering effects of the anesthetic or narcotics needed for pain relief. Fortunately, these factors usually diminish in the first few days to weeks following surgery.

Because there is nearly always some risk of temporary retention after an operation for stress incontinence, a catheter is commonly used to drain the bladder until tissue swelling decreases and the woman feels well enough to try urinating on her own. The catheter can be either a Foley catheter inserted through the urethra or a suprapubic catheter inserted during the operation through a small puncture in the abdomen.

The urethral Foley catheter has two advantages: it doesn't puncture the skin, and it doesn't require special procedures to remove it. It is best used after operations that have a high chance of the patient's being able to urinate on her own within a day or two of surgery; these operations include the Burch suspension and the Kelly plication. If a woman is unable to urinate after a urethral catheter is removed, there are three treatment options.

1. The catheter can be reinserted for a few days and then removed for another attempt at urination. However, inserting a Foley catheter requires a medical professional, so this option entails a return trip to the hospital or a visit to the doctor's office or an emergency room to have the catheter reinserted.
2. Certain medications can relax the urethra and permit urination to take place. In our experience, however, these medications are usually not strong enough to overcome the degree of obstruction that can occur immediately after stress incontinence operations.
3. Using the technique called clean intermittent self-catheterization, a woman can catheterize herself at regular intervals until normal urination returns. This technique is not difficult for most women, although it requires some instruction and practice to master. Some women find self-catheterization difficult to per-

form regardless of how hard they try to learn it. The technique can be extremely difficult or impossible if the tissues are swollen or painful after surgery, if a woman is overweight or older, or if a woman has difficulty finding the urethra or using her hands well.

For more complicated operations, such as sling procedures, or if there is concern that the patient may have trouble urinating for the first few days after a urethral Foley catheter is removed, a suprapubic catheter may be inserted into the bladder through the skin just above the pubic bone. The suprapubic catheter allows the urethral tissues to rest completely after the surgery and avoids self-catheterization immediately after the operation. When the patient first attempts to urinate on her own, the catheter remains as a safety valve. If the woman has trouble emptying, the catheter can simply be opened and the residual urine drained into a collection bag. Once urination has returned to normal, the catheter is removed, and the area where the catheter had been inserted will heal in a few days to two weeks, depending on the size of the opening. The woman is left with nothing more than a small scar that looks like a round spot, less than a quarter of an inch across. A suprapubic catheter is typically sewn into place during the operation and has to be removed by a medical professional. It is safe, however, and can remain in place for several weeks without causing any harm.

Difficulty with urination after stress incontinence operations should rarely last more than four weeks. A small number of people have difficulty urinating for a longer time. At some point, the patient and her doctor will have to decide whether to evaluate the degree of difficulty and whether to treat the problem. If you are having trouble urinating two months after a stress incontinence operation, you should consider undergoing an evaluation. Two simple tests evaluate postoperative urinary obstruction:

1. The *urinary flow rate test* uses a specialized instrument to measure how fast urine comes out of the bladder. The instrument traces the speed of urine flow on a piece of paper, similar to a

tracing of heart activity in an electrocardiogram. The instrument can automatically determine the fastest flow rate that occurred and the total amount of urine that was released. The doctor will also look at the pattern made by the tracing; an intermittent or "sawtooth" pattern is abnormal and suggests either an obstruction or a weak bladder.

2. The *residual volume test* measures the amount of urine left in the bladder after urination (the postvoid residual). The amount of residual urine volume can be determined by ultrasound, by placing a catheter into the bladder, or by calculating the difference between the amount put into the bladder via catheter and the amount emptied.

Ideally, the patient will have had the flow rate and residual volume tests performed before her operation, so that the difference after the operation can be easily evaluated.

In general, if a woman's ability to empty her bladder was fairly normal before a stress incontinence operation and she has trouble emptying afterward, the operation probably caused the urethra to become too tight. If the obstruction persists beyond two months, another operation will likely be required to relieve the obstruction. Fortunately, in most cases good urination can be restored without a return of the original incontinence. The scarring produced by the original operation usually provides enough support so that incontinence does not return. In a few cases, the new surgery weakens or injures the urethra, and some degree of incontinence returns or new problems develop.

Surgery to correct obstruction after a stress incontinence operation can be performed in one of two ways. First, for slings and similar operations, a vaginal approach can be used to divide the sling by cutting it in half across the middle or near the middle. The entire sling usually does not have to be removed. The operation has a low risk of complications and a short recovery time, and the risk of damage to or loss of function of the structures involved is usually not great. Second, for suspensions originally done through an abdominal incision, such as MMK and Burch suspensions, the scar itself must be divided.

Women who experience partial obstruction or urinary retention after stress incontinence surgery will probably need to see a specialist in a larger medical center for both the evaluation and for the additional surgery.

Some women with a small degree of obstruction and difficulty urinating after stress incontinence surgery decide to tolerate the new problems as a minor nuisance, especially if they now have the desired relief from incontinence. Moreover, depending on the extent of urethral weakness and bladder dysfunction before the operation, a perfect result may not be possible after a stress incontinence operation. Nonetheless, the overall result may be a significant improvement in quality of life, and some women may not wish to risk possible damage to it.

*Kerri, 56 years old, had been experiencing incontinence for four years. At first, only very strenuous activity produced a small amount of leakage, and she was satisfied with using a small liner to absorb the liquid. Gradually, the leakage worsened to the point that it frequently occurred when she did undemanding activities, including leisurely walking. Kerri used several large pads each day and was always fearful of having a bad episode in public. Most distressing of all to Kerri was her new reluctance to attend dance evenings, which for years had been a large part of her and her husband's social life. When she finally decided to consult her doctor, the doctor diagnosed weak support for the vaginal wall and bladder neck. With this information, Kerri decided to undergo a Burch procedure to suspend the bladder neck.*

*After the procedure, Kerri had no incontinence, but she did have difficulty emptying her bladder. She knew this was a possibility for several days after the operation, but the problem persisted for weeks. She also began to have recurrent bladder infections, and she complained of frequency and urgency. She returned to her doctor for an evaluation and had a urine flow rate test that showed obstructed flow. The doctor determined that the bladder neck suspension was too tight and was obstructing the urethra. Kerri was referred to a specialist interested in women's urology at a large center specializing in urology. The specialist proposed two options: using clean intermittent self-catheterization indefinitely, or un-*

*dergoing a urethrolysis to free the urethra. The urethrolysis procedure involved an abdominal operation to release the scar tissue. Kerri decided she was willing to accept the risk that her incontinence would return so that she wouldn't have to use self-catheterization permanently. She had the urethrolysis, and the procedure successfully eliminated her difficulty in urinating. The bladder infections, urgency, and frequency also stopped. Kerri's incontinence did recur to a small degree with strenuous physical activity, but for most activities she is dry. She resumed dancing and wears a liner when she dances, but most of the time wearing a liner is unnecessary.*

## Persistent or Recurrent Incontinence

One of the most frustrating experiences after surgical treatment for stress incontinence is to find that you still have urine leakage. The amount or frequency of leakage may be less than it was before but still a nuisance. It may be completely unchanged or — the most feared complication — it may even be worse. There are many possible reasons for persistent leakage after stress incontinence surgery: the operation was not performed properly, the wrong kind of operation was done for the type of incontinence, the operation depended on tissues too weak to hold stitches, or the preoperative evaluation missed some aspects of bladder dysfunction, such as bladder overactivity or overflow incontinence. Occasionally, a fistula may form.

After the initial surprise and disappointment of continued incontinence, the best thing to do is to return to a doctor for another evaluation. The evaluation will most likely require a bladder (urodynamic) test and a cystoscopic examination and possibly an imaging study. The additional stress and strain of dealing with a bad result and the additional treatment required to overcome it can drain your personal resources. Nevertheless, it is always worthwhile having another evaluation to find out exactly what the situation is. You should then have the necessary information to make a decision about further treatment.

Unless the problem is severe bladder dysfunction, further treatment often successfully addresses persistent incontinence. However, a woman must consider how far she is willing to go to achieve a good result. If the continued leakage represents a significant improvement over the previous situation, she may decide to tolerate the leakage. For example, a woman who previously required three to four larger absorbent pads per day and could not participate in physical exercise or social events now finds that she can do these things even though she still requires one smaller pad per day. Depending on the results of her postoperative evaluation, her options could be to reject further treatment and continue using the single pad per day; have a collagen injection to provide further improvement, albeit temporarily; or repeat the surgery. She may decide to try collagen injections initially and undergo a second operation later on.

If the leakage is unchanged or worse after an operation, the new evaluation should determine whether any of the initial causes of incontinence are still contributing to the problem or whether new causes have arisen. Again, depending on the results of the evaluation, both surgical and nonsurgical options may be available. The patient will have to reevaluate her goals and decide whether she is willing to continue pursuing surgical treatment.

Sometimes, preexisting or newly occurring bladder dysfunction is the cause of persistent incontinence after surgery. If the leakage results from bladder overactivity, unwanted bladder contractions or spasms are strong enough to overcome the effects of the stress incontinence operation and force urine through the urethra. Medication to relax bladder overactivity may help in this situation. However, medication may also relax the bladder too much so that, because of the surgically improved urethra or bladder neck, the bladder can't contract sufficiently to force urine through the urethra. In this case, a woman will be unable to empty her bladder and will need to perform clean intermittent self-catheterization. Another bladder dysfunction that can cause leakage is overflow incontinence, which results from poor bladder sensation or weak bladder contraction. Even when a stress incontinence operation is properly performed and the repair is sound, overflow incontinence can occur. Urethral support may be good, but the muscles of the urethra itself are not strong enough to withstand increasing bladder pressure as the volume rises and the urethral walls are simply pushed apart by the growing volume of urine. A person in this situation can use clean intermittent self-catheterization to empty the bladder and manage the problem, but if this was not the expected result, a neurourologist should be consulted.

## Urinary Tract Infection

Urinary tract infections are common in women; many women will experience at least one, usually shortly after becoming sexually active. The typical symptoms of a urinary tract infection include urgency, frequency, and pain or burning on urination, and some women also occasionally have blood in the urine, fever, or chills. The symptoms usually respond quickly to a short course of antibiotics. Simple urinary infection is most common in a woman's younger years when her urethra is shorter and she is having early sexual experiences, decreases somewhat during middle age, and increases again as she grows older and passes through menopause with the associated changes that reduce her resistance to infection.

Women with incontinence may have a slightly increased tendency toward urinary tract infection because of the constant dampness near the opening of the urethra. Bacteria grow more easily in a moist environment, and from the urethral opening they have only a short distance to travel to infect the urine in the bladder. Successful treatment of incontinence may reduce the number of urinary infections a woman experiences.

In general, surgical treatment for stress incontinence should not make urinary tract infections more likely or increase their frequency. However, vulnerability to infections can increase temporarily after an operation simply because catheters have been inserted into the bladder and normal tissue-healing mechanisms that protect against infection are temporarily disrupted. Basically, a person's defenses are down for a short time after an operation.

If urinary infection develops after stress incontinence surgery or doesn't go away despite antibiotic treatment, there are a few possible causes to investigate. The first is the presence of a foreign object in the urinary tract. For example, sutures may have penetrated the bladder during the operation or worked their way through the bladder or urethral walls, an artificial material used for a sling may have eroded through the urethra or bladder, or part of a catheter may have broken off and still be in the bladder. Any foreign object in the bladder can serve as the base, or seed, for the formation of a stone because urine contains a variety of minerals such as calcium and phosphate that can adhere to and build up around an object. Urinary tract stones can usually be identified by ultrasound, and occasionally by X-ray, and a cystoscopic examination will confirm their presence. A stone may also cause pain in the bladder or the lower part of the abdomen and pelvis; some women with urinary stones experience pain and bleeding during urination. A urinary stone can usually be treated successfully with minor surgery that may involve inserting an instrument through the urethra to crush and remove the stone or removing the stone through a small suprapubic incision in the bladder. Laser treatment can also be used, as with kidney stones. Sometimes, artificial material in the urinary tract will cause a urinary infection, as well as possible pain and bleeding, even before a stone forms.

Another reason for persistent or recurrent urinary tract infections following incontinence surgery is the presence of residual urine in the bladder. An obstructed or weak bladder that can't empty completely increases a woman's risk of infection because the urine spends more time in the bladder and bacteria from the rectum can move along the perineum and up the urethra to colonize the residual urine. Addressing the cause of residual urine generally eliminates infection, as does taking a low dose of antibiotics on a regular basis to prevent bacteria from colonizing and increasing in number. Sometimes, the cause of infection has nothing to do with the incontinence operation, and in this case the woman is treated just as anyone else with urinary infection in her age group would be treated.

## Development of a Fistula

A fistula is an abnormal passage or open connection between two organs or structures in the body or between an organ or structure inside the body and the skin. Women in the industrialized world most commonly develop a fistula between the vagina and the bladder, termed a vesicovaginal fistula (Figure 28), after a hysterectomy. In

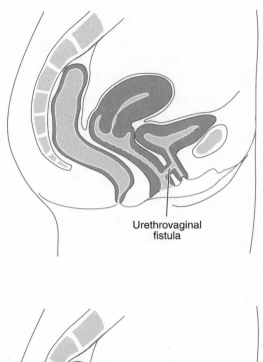

Urethrovaginal
fistula

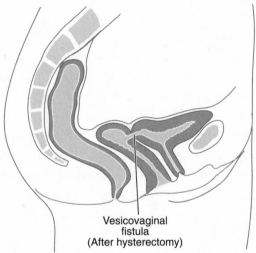

Vesicovaginal
fistula
(After hysterectomy)

Figure 28. Urethrovaginal and vesicovaginal fistulas

this case, removal of the uterus leaves an opening at the top of the vagina where the cervix had been. Although the vagina is sewn shut after a hysterectomy, the vagina and bladder are close to each other within the pelvis, and a fistula can develop if the tissues are under tension or are weakened by the surgery. The vagina-to-bladder fistula allows urine to pass from the bladder to the vagina and leak out the vaginal opening 24 hours a day. An operation is required to fix the problem.

After an incontinence operation, a urethrovaginal fistula can develop because of poor wound healing, infection, or a breakdown of the tissues separating the urinary tract from the vagina. A fistula may also develop if an artificial sling erodes through the urethra and the vagina, leaving a space where it passed. If the fistula develops at or above the level of the urethral sphincter, the woman will experience urinary leakage 24 hours a day, just like a woman with a posthysterectomy fistula. Most women with a fistula in this position want to have it repaired. If the fistula is located farther down on the urethra, the woman will most likely remain continent, but she will experience a double or spraying stream during urination. Some women tolerate the spraying urination if it doesn't cause them too much trouble, while others opt to have the fistula surgically repaired.

*Gloria, a 62-year-old primary school teacher, had a hysterectomy because of heavy bleeding. She had not had any symptoms of incontinence, despite having given birth to four children. During the hysterectomy operation, Gloria's bladder was torn very slightly as it was pushed off the cervix to complete the hysterectomy. However, the bladder injury was so slight that it wasn't noticed immediately.*

*Gloria started noticing some increased discharge and constant wetness within four weeks of the surgical procedure. She went to see her surgeon, who diagnosed the presence of a fistula between the bladder and vagina, most likely the result of the minor bladder tear during the hysterectomy. Gloria insisted that the fistula be corrected immediately. The surgeon used a vaginal approach to separate the bladder and vaginal wall and close the defect. Gloria did well initially but started noticing a recurrence of her symptoms after about two months. Once again, she returned to the surgeon, who reevaluated her and found that part of the fistula remained. For the second fistula repair, the surgeon made a pad from a piece of tissue removed from Gloria's labia, the lips at the opening of the vagina. The second repair held, and Gloria has not had further incontinence symptoms.*

# Erosion or Infection from Synthetic Materials

Synthetic materials are used in some slings, as well as in urethral sphincter cuffs. When the synthetic material presses on natural tissue, it can make a hole through the tissue and work its way out to the skin or into another compartment of the body. The erosion may occur immediately after an operation, or it may be delayed by as long as several years. This type of erosion by a synthetic material can cause infection and lead to permanent problems. Erosion or infection from synthetic materials is a serious complication that requires surgical treatment and frequently causes difficulty in long-term repair. Almost all synthetic materials previously used for slings have turned out to have a high erosion rate, so surgeons have been cautious about using these materials in the vaginal area. They're still used in some cases, such as a cystocele repair. However, one recently developed synthetic material called tension-free vaginal tape (TVT) appears to have a lower erosion rate. TVT has been available for about eleven years, so its erosion risk continues to be monitored.

Once a synthetic material reaches a urine-containing compartment of the body or works its way out to the skin, infection is inevitable because there are always bacteria in the urethra and on the skin surface. The infection can then spread along the rest of the synthetic material inside the body, causing further internal infection and tissue damage. Infection is a serious problem that must be taken care of as soon as it is discovered, and the synthetic material in contact with urine or skin must be removed as soon as possible. The tissue can then be allowed to heal, and the person's condition can be reassessed afterward. Synthetic materials can also become infected before they erode natural tissues, with localized pain often being the only symptom of the infection. At times, there may also be a mass of swollen, infected tissue or a draining sinus close to the infected tissues. A draining sinus is a cavity in the abdomen or vaginal area that fills with pus or urine and then drains to the outside of the body by whatever pathway is easiest for it to follow.

As the following two case studies illustrate, the damage caused by synthetic materials can sometimes be successfully repaired, but at other times related problems and incontinence symptoms persist.

Rhonda, 54 years old, had been using two large pads per day for about three years when she underwent the placement of a synthetic sling. The surgery went well, and she recovered quickly. Her incontinence symptoms had been completely eliminated. She was delighted with the result and found herself with extra energy that she put into looking after her baby granddaughter three days a week. Two months after the sling operation, she began having bloody vaginal spotting. Initially, her doctor told her that the vaginal incision from the operation was healing, but another month passed and there was no improvement.

When Rhonda returned to the doctor, she examined the vagina and discovered that the edges of the sling had eroded the vaginal wall and were exposed to the vaginal canal. Rhonda had a second operation to remove the sling and the sutures that had held it in place. The eroded vaginal wall was left to heal on its own, which is the usual practice. Three weeks later, Rhonda returned to the doctor for a follow-up vaginal examination, which showed that the eroded portion of the vagina had healed. Because of the scar tissue that had formed in the space occupied by the sling, Rhonda's urethra remained well supported, and she experienced only rare leakage episodes.

Margaret, 47 years old, had a synthetic sling operation for leakage that was causing her to wear three large pads a day. Two days after the operation, she experienced significant pain on the right side of her back. She was nauseated, and her blood pressure started going up. An ultrasound examination in the hospital showed that her right kidney was blocked. She was taken back to the operating room, where the surgeon discovered that the sling had pierced through the urethra and bladder and had moved all the way over to block the entrance of the right ureter into the bladder. The extensive movement of the sling had probably happened so quickly because there had been too much tension and the nearby tissues were weakened by the operation. The surgeon removed the sling immediately and placed a short tube called a stent in the ureter to splint it during the healing process. A suprapubic catheter placed into the bladder by a puncture in the lower abdominal wall drained the bladder.

One month later, the ureter had healed, and the stent was removed. However, the injury to the urethra and bladder from the sling meant that

*Margaret's bladder was now small and overactive. The urethra was weak, which had been the reason for the initial sling operation. Margaret was faced with both stress and urge incontinence. She resumed using absorbent pads, and she tried various medications for the bladder overactivity. Margaret eventually underwent another sling operation, this time using a sling made from her own thigh tissue. This second sling operation was successful in stopping her stress incontinence. However, her bladder capacity remained small, and her bladder continued to be overactive. Despite large doses of medication, Margaret continues to require two medium to large pads a day because of urge incontinence due to bladder overactivity.*

## Persistent or New-Onset Urgency or Urge Incontinence

Some women experience both stress and urge incontinence, termed *mixed incontinence*. As discussed in Chapter 3, the presence of urine flowing into a weakened urethra during increases in intra-abdominal pressure may stimulate the feeling of having to urinate, which gives rise to the feeling of urgency. The woman may feel like she can't "hold it," she may experience a sudden urge to urinate when she stands up or gets out of bed, or she may just frequently have the feeling that she has to empty her bladder. Many women who experience urgency with stress incontinence obtain excellent relief after successful treatment of the stress incontinence. It is not clear why treating the stress incontinence eliminates the urge incontinence, but it may have to do with a tighter or better supported urethra preventing urine from reaching the sensitive part of the urethra that triggers the urination reflex.

Not all women with mixed incontinence get relief from urgency and urge incontinence after stress incontinence treatment, though. In these women, the urgency may be due to problems that are not related to urethral weakness. For example, there may be difficulty with the nerves supplying sensation and contraction signals to the bladder, leading to symptoms of overactive bladder. When this kind of urgency exists, successfully treating the stress incontinence will not correct the urgency. The urgency that remains after surgery may occur in no more than 15 percent of people with mixed incontinence who undergo surgery, but it can be a serious enough problem that the benefits of being rid of the stress incontinence seem minor in comparison.

About 10 to 15 percent of people undergoing stress incontinence operations may develop urgency when none was present before. The urgency may or may not be associated with urge incontinence, and the severity of the urgency varies. Urgency can develop after surgery if the repair has made the urethra too tight. The bladder's efforts to overcome the increased resistance may lead to changes in nerve and muscle function of the bladder, generating urgency symptoms and possibly also an overactive bladder. Most people can tolerate mild urgency for a few months after stress incontinence surgery. If necessary, medications such as Ditropan or Detrol can be prescribed. If the urgency is severe or associated with urge incontinence, however, further testing should be considered. In particular, a doctor will evaluate the patient for possible obstruction, infection, erosion, and presence of a foreign object, all of which can make the bladder overreact to small stimuli.

## Obstructed Kidney

The ureters, which carry urine from the kidneys to the bladder, enter the bladder in an area close to where stress incontinence operations take place. As a result, injuries to the ureters, although rare, are possible during stress incontinence operations. Although there are standard methods for making sure that the ureters are open before the patient leaves the operating room, they can sometimes become blocked. A ureter may be partially or totally blocked by suture material, a sling, or other foreign material. Too much tension on the tissues surrounding the ureters can also deform one or both of the ureters, leading to a partial or total blockage of the ureter and kidney. If a kidney is completely blocked for three weeks, it will permanently lose function. If it is partially blocked, it may take much longer to lose function, the kidney may become infected, or stones may develop. Any one of these situations is undesirable, so an obstructed kidney should be identified as soon as possible. As long as treatment begins quickly, most injuries to a ureter can be repaired without permanent loss of kidney function.

A blocked kidney can be identified by a variety of symptoms. A woman may experience pain along the side of her body or in the abdomen due to the blocked kidney's increased efforts to overcome the obstruction. A person's blood pressure may rise temporarily shortly after obstruction of a kidney. Finally, there may be a temporary rise in the amount of waste products — measured by one protein product called creatinine — in the blood. The sudden rise in creatinine indicates that one kidney has suddenly stopped functioning. Sometimes the signs and symptoms of an obstructed kidney will not be apparent right after surgery. For example, a suture or a clip may wear a hole through a ureter a few days or even weeks after surgery. In this case, urine may start to leak inside the abdomen, where it will accumulate. Again, this is a rare but serious complication that requires immediate attention to drain the urine and repair the ureter.

Though it seems logical, monitoring the urine output after surgery will not help to identify the presence of one blocked kidney. Because most people have two kidneys, blocking only one kidney will not lead to a decrease in urine production.

## New Pain

Operations for stress incontinence do not usually produce much pain and almost never lead to chronic pain unless there were significant problems with the operation itself. In the immediate postoperative period, pain may indicate a wound infection or obstructed kidney. If the operation was complicated by bleeding or if there was scar tissue from previous operations, the wound from the most recent operation may heal with new internal scars that bind structures together and result in pain. If a sling or suspension is too tight, pressure on the bladder during urination can lead to pain. If a foreign object such as a synthetic sling or bone anchor was used and has become infected, the infection itself may cause pain. Except for a reasonable amount of discomfort from the surgery itself in the first few days and weeks after the operation, new pain after surgery should be considered an abnormal complication and should be investigated.

The complications described in this chapter are not inevitable ones, but they are possible, and you should be aware of them and how they can be addressed before deciding on the treatment you wish to pursue. Don't dwell on these complications. As we recap in Chapter 10, your best chance for both short-term and long-term success is to gather as much information as you can, choose an experienced doctor, ask questions, and make a careful decision about your treatment.

# ℐ 10 ℐ

## *Summary:*

## *Taking Control of Urinary Incontinence*

We hope that by reading all or parts of this book you will have gained a better understanding of urinary incontinence, its causes, the possible ways to deal with or treat it, and the types of information you need to discuss with your doctor. Briefly, we would like to summarize the key points that we advocate for every woman dealing with urinary incontinence, no matter how slight or how severe the symptoms.

- **Don't suffer in silence.**

    You are not alone in your struggle with incontinence. Many, many women experience incontinence, and it is not necessary to deal with it in isolation. Numerous health professionals are available to help you control or treat your incontinence.

- **Find the right doctor for you.**

    The relationship you build with your doctor is extremely important for you to feel comfortable as a partner in your health care. You need to find a physician who listens to your concerns and takes time to answer your questions, in addition to being knowledgeable and experienced in his or her field. If you feel uncomfortable or uncertain about how well you and your doctor can communicate, consider looking for another doctor. Ask family members and friends for a recommendation, search the Internet or yellow pages for an alternative, or speak with a nurse or other allied health care worker at a local public health facility.

It's all right to switch to another doctor if you think your needs will be better met.

- **Be an active partner in your health care.**

For the best possible outcome, you need to become an active partner in your health care. This means doing a little research — reading this book, for example — and gaining an understanding of your particular situation. Learn as much as possible about the symptoms, condition, and causes of your incontinence.

Ask questions of your doctor at every step: during evaluation and medical testing, during the discussions about treatment options, during treatment itself, and during follow-up sessions.

Finally, tell your doctor everything relevant to your condition. Every piece of information that you share with the doctor will help him or her diagnose your incontinence and, importantly, suggest appropriate options for you to consider.

- **Evaluate your priorities and goals.**

Determine what you want to achieve with incontinence management or treatment and what success looks like for you. What is important in your life at the moment? Perhaps a noninvasive treatment would be acceptable even if it provides only temporary relief from your symptoms. You can always pursue other options when or if circumstances change later on. When evaluating your goals, keep in mind that a complete cure may be unrealistic, so you may have to make some compromises.

- **Learn about the many options available to manage and treat incontinence.**

You can select a therapy that is completely noninvasive or one that is only minimally invasive. If you wish, you can start by trying to manage your symptoms and move to more aggressive treatment only if the symptoms worsen. Many women use absorbent pads and other similar products indefinitely and find they are able to live full, active lives without pursuing any further incontinence options.

- **Don't assume that surgery is the best or only route to take.**

Numerous options are available for treating incontinence. Surgery may be a good option in your situation, but there may also be more conservative or minimally invasive options that could work well. Find out about all options and evaluate the benefits and risks of each as you make your decision.

- **Take time to make decisions.**

    Don't be in a rush to make a decision, because there may be a lot at stake for you in terms of recovery time or possible complications. Consider all available options before deciding which to pursue, and try not to be swayed by the treatment that a friend or family member had: every person has a slightly different situation, so not all treatments are appropriate in all cases. Don't be afraid to get a second opinion if it helps you make a sound decision. Particularly with surgical procedures, the best incontinence treatment in terms of providing good, long-term results is usually the first one you undergo.

- **Build a support network of family and friends, or join a support group.**

    It can be hard to talk about personal health issues that are as embarrassing as incontinence can be. Yet for many women talking about such problems provides both reassurance and information. If you don't have family or friends you feel comfortable confiding in, there are many other people in the community to whom you can turn. For example, speak with a counselor or contact your local health center to ask about support groups. By joining a support group, you will find women in situations similar to yours with whom you can share your fears and concerns, as well as your triumphs when you find a successful option for your incontinence.

# Glossary

**Allograft**

Graft of living human tissue obtained from a donor who is not the person for whom the graft is to be used (as opposed to an autograft, which is taken from the person for whom it is to be used).

**Anesthetic, general**

A state of pain control, management, and monitoring provided for patients undergoing medical procedures, usually supervised by a professional such as an anesthesiologist or nurse anesthetist and involving the patient's going to sleep with airway control. When most people think about "going to sleep" for an operation, they are thinking about general anesthesia.

**Anesthetic, local**

A blocking of the nerves in a specific area of the body by the injection of medications or by the application of medications to the skin (surface administration) without the patient's going to sleep. An example is when a dentist injects an area of the mouth with medication to "numb" the area before a dental procedure. Cystoscopy is commonly performed with surface (topical) placement of an anesthetic lubricant.

**Bladder**

A hollow, rounded organ for the storage and expulsion of urine, located behind the pubic bone of the lower front of the pelvis.

**Bladder diverticulum**

A cystic pouch or cavity resulting from a defect in the musculature of the bladder wall that may store urine and inhibit normal bladder function. Can also cause stones and infection.

**Bladder neck**

The tapered lower portion of the bladder that funnels into the urethra to permit expulsion of urine. Normally closed at rest, it starts to widen and give way to intra-abdominal pressure as vaginal support or intrinsic musculature begins to weaken in stress incontinence.

**Bowel**

The long tubular organ that extends from the mouth to the rectum and guides and expels food from ingestion to expulsion. Two portions of the bowel, the large bowel (colon) and small bowel (jejunum and ileum), can be used in the reconstruction of the urinary tract.

**Catheter**

A thin, hollow, flexible tube made of plastic, silicon, or similar material, used to drain urine out of the bladder. Can be inserted periodically by the patient through the urethra, left in for a short period of time after a procedure or longer (indwelling), or used as a long-term drainage option for the bladder when placed into it through the skin (suprapubic).

**Connective tissue**

Elastic and sinewy components of the body that link structures and fill empty spaces.

**Cystocele**

An area of vaginal weakness involving part of the bladder wall. On examination, a cystocele usually appears as an asymptomatic bulge in the vagina or a more advanced visible protrusion of the vagina. May or may not be associated with incontinence.

**Cystometrogram**

The recorded tracing of pressure and volume relationships in the bladder during filling from an external fluid source. Usually part of the clinical testing of bladder function, often followed by a flow rate test, a residual volume estimate, and cystoscopy.

**Cystoscopy**

Clinical examination of the interior of the bladder and urethra performed with a thin, hollow tube (the endoscope, or cystoscope) equipped with a lens, water for filling, and a light source for viewing.

**Cystourethrocele**

A weakened or "relaxed" area of the vagina similar to a cystocele but extending low enough to include the urethra as part of the relaxed area or protrusion.

**Diverticulum**

See Bladder diverticulum; Urethral diverticulum.

**Embolus**

A blood clot (termed a *thrombus*) that breaks away from the site of its development and travels to another site to produce blockage. Pulmonary emboli, for example, are clots that have broken off and traveled to the lung. Embolic strokes result from similar fragments of clot that enter the brain's arterial circulation. *See also* Thrombus.

**Endoscope**

A hollow, tubular instrument used to inspect internal structures through small openings in the body. Examples are a cystoscope (introduced through the urethra) and a laparoscope (introduced into the abdominal cavity through a puncture in the body wall).

**Enterocele**

A weak area of the vagina involving the upper part of the vaginal wall. On examination, it usually appears as an asymptomatic bulge in the vagina or a more advanced visible protrusion of the vagina. It may also appear as the uterus and cervix descending into the vagina, or the vaginal remnant (scar left after the cervix is removed) after a hysterectomy. Some bowel may often be located just under the vaginal surface of the enterocele. Usually not associated with incontinence, although it is commonly associated with other vagina hernias or protrusions.

**Enuresis**

Bedwetting. A term specifically used to indicate wetting at night. Normal in infants and young children. Typically stops by age 5, although in some children it may persist into adolescence. A small percentage of adults have primary enuresis, though when it comes on later in life, it is almost always a cardinal sign of problems with the lower urinary tract.

**Epidural**

A kind of regional anesthesia (anesthesia directed at a specific part of the body to block the nerves only in that area) administered through a small catheter placed by needle into the back, just outside the location of the nerve roots of the spinal cord. Medication can be administered to achieve a desired level of relief from the waist down (typically) during or after a procedure. Frequently used to achieve pain relief without muscle paralysis in labor and delivery and for longer operations or those in which administration of pain relief may be required for several days afterward.

**Episiotomy**

A surgically created incision to widen the entrance of the birth canal during delivery. Closed after delivery. It is done to reduce or prevent uncontrolled vaginal tears, but its role in preventing long-term damage to the perineum remains controversial.

**Fibroid**

A benign smooth-muscle tumor of the uterus.

**Fistula**

Abnormal passage or opening between two normally separate hollow structures. Examples are a vesicovaginal fistula (connection between the bladder and the vagina), which may occur after hysterectomy; a urethrovaginal fistula (between the urethra and the vagina), which can occur after prolonged labor or urethral diverticulum surgery, and an enterovesical fistula (between the bowel and the bladder), which can occur in advanced diverticulosis or diverticulitis. The first two lead to urinary leakage, the third to chronic infection and passage of air with urine.

**Foley catheter**

A catheter kept in place by an inflatable internal balloon at its tip.

**Homograft**

A graft taken from the person for whom it is to be used.

**Hysterectomy**

Surgical removal of the uterus for benign or malignant conditions. It can be performed by a vaginal approach (no obvious incision) or an abdominal approach, with or without laparoscopic assistance. A total hysterectomy usually means removal of the uterus with the ovaries; a subtotal hysterectomy means that the ovaries were left. Some hysterectomies can be performed abdominally without removing the cervix (supracervical hysterectomy). Vaginal hysterectomy requires removal of the cervix.

**Interstitial cystitis**

A painful inflammatory condition of the bladder more common in women than men, often associated with pelvic pain and frequent urgent voiding. Sometimes associated with a small-capacity, contracted bladder with a lining that may crack and bleed during filling.

**Laparoscope**

A surgical endoscope introduced into the abdominal cavity through a puncture in the body wall. Some instruments contain a camera for viewing, and others contain surgical instruments for manipulation.

**Mixed incontinence**

A term used to describe symptoms of both urgency and stress urinary incontinence.

**MRI**

Magnetic resonance imaging. A method of advanced three-dimensional imaging that does not require X-rays or iodinated contrast but cannot be used with people who have magnetic pieces of metal within their body.

**Nocturia**

The symptom of waking at night in order to urinate. It usually implies that a person will awaken and get to the toilet, as opposed to people who wet the bed or wake up already wet with a feeling that they need to void or an awareness of voiding.

**Overactive bladder**

A term used to describe the symptom complex of frequent and urgent voiding, with or without incontinence.

**Overflow incontinence**

A type of leakage resulting from a weak urethra and reduced bladder sensation or bladder emptying (or both), with leakage of urine commonly occurring at a bladder capacity that would lead a person who doesn't have this condition to empty his or her bladder.

**Pelvic floor**

The muscles and soft tissues that form the support for the bottom of the abdominal cavity.

**Pelvic nerve**

The final common pathway of nerves from the spinal cord that travel to the bladder.

**Perineum**

The tissue bridging the back of the vagina to the rectum, often stretched or surgically cut (episiotomy) during childbirth.

**Pessary**

A medical device placed in the vagina to block motion and herniation by supporting the vaginal wall.

**Prolapse**

Condition in which an organ falls out of its normal position. In a vaginal prolapse, the vaginal wall and/or the uterus protrudes through the vagina, with an intra-abdominal structure frequently behind it.

**Pubic bone**

The front part of the pelvic bone, which can be felt through the skin.

**Pudendal nerve**

The final common pathway for motor and sensory nerves traveling to and from voluntary muscles in the pelvis, including the urethral sphincter.

**Rectocele**

An area of vaginal weakness involving the back wall associated with a protrusion of rectum behind it.

**Rectum**

The last few inches of the large bowel, storing solid waste until it is eliminated from the body.

**Sling procedure**

An operation providing direct support to the urethra using a natural or synthetic strap (sling). In contrast, other operations provide indirect support to the urethra.

**Smooth muscle**

Muscle that is not under voluntary control, such as bowel, bladder, and urinary tract muscles.

**Speculum**

An instrument inserted into the vagina to permit direct visual inspection of the cervix.

**Stoma**

An opening in the abdominal wall, usually created surgically. Opening of an internal structure onto the abdominal wall, such as a urinary stoma.

**Straight catheter**

A catheter without a balloon, usually used for intermittent catheterization or a one-time drainage of the bladder.

**Stress incontinence**

Involuntary loss of urine under conditions of physical stress that lead to increases in intra-abdominal pressure. May be due to vaginal weakness, urethral weakness, or both.

**Striated muscle**

In contrast to smooth and cardiac muscle, a kind of muscle that is under voluntary control, such as the urethral sphincter.

**Suprapubic catheter**

A catheter placed into the bladder by a puncture or surgical incision in the abdominal wall.

**Suspension procedure**

A kind of operation for stress incontinence that supports the urethra by attaching the vagina near the urethra to other nearby structures to reduce movement during stress.

**Suture**

Surgical thread, either absorbable or permanent, natural or synthetic, woven or monofilament, provided in different sizes and attached to different kinds of needles.

**Thrombus**

A blood clot leading to blockage. Deep vein thrombosis, a potentially serious medical condition, is the formation of a blood clot in a deep vein, such as the deep veins of the leg.

**Ureter**

A hollow, thin muscular tube conducting urine from kidney to bladder. Runs close to the cervix and ovary and can be injured during gynecological or stress incontinence operations.

**Urethra**

The narrow muscular tube 2–3 inches long that allows urine to pass from the bladder to the outside of the body.

**Urethral diverticulum**

A cystic pouch or balloon projecting off the main urethral channel, usually caused by chronic infection that has damaged the surrounding tissue and resulting in local pain (pain in that specific area), pressure, difficulty with sexual activity, and leakage of urine.

**Urethral sphincter**

The structures forming the natural closure of the urethra to prevent involuntary loss of urine.

**Urethrocele**

Like a cystourethrocele, but the vaginal defect is more limited to the area immediately in front of the urethra and bladder neck. See also Cystourethrocele.

**Urethroscopy**

Examination of the urethra using an endoscope.

**Urge incontinence**

Involuntary loss of urine that is preceded by a strong feeling of having to void and that cannot be stopped.

**Urinalysis**

Chemical and microscopic examination of the urine to look for blood, infection, signs of renal disease (protein), or diabetes.

**Urinary retention**

Inability to empty the bladder. May be total or partial, may be painful or silent.

**Urodynamic test**

A general term used to describe the combination of tests for evaluating the function of the lower tract and urethral competence. Usually includes a cystometrogram, a flow rate and residual volume estimate, and determination of leak point pressures or urethral closure pressures and muscle function.

**Uterus**

The hollow, smooth muscular organ that forms the womb.

**Vagina**

The birth canal.

**Vulva**

The external female genitalia.

**Xenograft**

Graft taken from another animal species for implantation into humans.

# Resources

*The following list of resources, by no means exhaustive, provides the names of organizations and groups from which you can obtain further information about incontinence, finding a doctor, incontinence products, newsletters, and support groups.*

**American Urogynecological Society**
www.augs.org

**American Urological Association**
www.urologyhealth.org/
A Web site written by urologists for patients.
The site has a search function to find a urologist
(www.urologyhealth.org/find_urologist/).

**American Urological Association Foundation**
1000 Corporate Boulevard
Linthicum, MD 21090
866-746-4282
www.auafoundation.org/auafhome.asp

**International Continence Society**
www.icsoffice.org
The Web site has a link to www.continenceworldwode.org.

**Medline Plus**
www.nlm.nih.gov/medlineplus/encyclopedia.html
An encyclopedia of medical terms and conditions.

**National Association for Continence**

800-252-3337

www.nafc.org

NAFC publishes a resource book of incontinence products each year. The Web site has a function to do a Specialist Search.

**National Association for Home Care and Hospice**

www.nahc.org/famcaregiver.html

**National Institutes of Health**

9000 Rockville Pike

Bethesda, MD 20892

301-496-4000

www.nih.gov

The Web site lists hotline phone numbers for information on various health issues (www.nih.gov/health/infoline.htm).

**National Kidney and Urologic Diseases Information Clearinghouse**

3 Information Way

Bethesda, MD 20892-3580

800-891-5390

http://kidney.niddk.nih.gov/

On the Web site, use the search terms "Urinary Incontinence in Women" and "Bladder Control for Women Campaign" to find relevant information.

**National Women's Health Information Center**

Department of Health and Human Services

8270 Willow Oaks Corporate Drive

Fairfax, VA 22031

800-994-9662

www.4woman.gov

**National Women's Health Resource Center**

www.healthywomen.org/

**Simon Foundation for Continence**

PO Box 815

Wilmette, IL 60091

800-237-4666

www.simonfoundation.org

The Web site has an online database of incontinence products, titled Incontinence Solutions.

**Society of Gynecologic Surgeons**

PO Box 381063

Germantown, TN 38183-1063

901-682-2079

www.sgsonline.org/

Search for a gynecologist by selecting "Find an SGS Physician."

# Index

Page numbers in **boldface** type refer to figures.

Abdominal pressure, 17–19, 29, 93, 158

Absorbent pads, 68–71, **69**

Age: incontinence and, 1, 2, 3, 19, 39–41; at menopause, 31

Allografts, 108, 110, 165; of cadaver tissue, 108–9

American Urogynecologic Society, 173

American Urological Association, 173

American Urological Association Foundation, 173

Anal sphincter, 53, 54

Anesthesia: for collagen injections, 89, 90; for cystoscopy, 63; epidural, 100, 167; general, 63–64, 96, 105, 165; for InterStim implantation, 115; local, 63, 106, 115, 165; saddle, 36; for sling operations, 105–6; spinal, 96, 100, 105; for suspension operations, 96, 101

Antibiotics, 43, 58, 62, 65, 121, 142

Artificial urinary sphincter, 113–14, **114**

Augmentation cystoplasty, 118–20, **119**

"Bashful" bladder, 57

Becoming a partner in your care, 45–46, 125–26, 163

Bedside commode, 41

Bedwetting, 20, 38–39, 87, 167

Biofeedback, 77–82, **79, 81,** 134, 139

Bladder, 7, **8,** 9–10, **13, 14, 28,** 165; augmentation of, 118–20, **119,** 137; "bashful," 57; control of, 15; diverticulum of, 165; infection of, 20, 22, 27; overactive, 21–22, 41, 87, 151, 169; overstretching of, 98; in pregnancy, 22–23; pressure in, 10; spasms of, 35, 137, 151

Bladder cycle, 13–14, **14**

Bladder diary, 49, **50**

Bladder neck, **8,** 9, 10, 165; kinking of, **27**

Bladder test, 56, 58–62, **60**

Bladder-training biofeedback, 78–80, 82

Bowel, 166

Brain: control of muscles by, 12–13, 15; stroke, injury, or tumor of, 33–35; urinary tract and, 33–34, **34**

Bricker urinary diversion, 116–18, **117**

Bulking agents, injectable, 63, 88–93, **90**

Burch vaginal suspension, 96, 102–3, **103,** 123, 146, 148

Cadaver grafts, 108–9
Carbon-coated latex rubber particle injections (Dura-Sphere), 92
Catheter, 59, 73, 166; Foley, 31, 73–74, 98, 106, 121, 128–29, 146, 147, 168; indwelling, 74, 140; straight, 73, 98, 121, **122,** 170; suprapubic, 74, 106, 146, 147, 170; urination after removal of, 97–98
Catheterization: clean intermittent self-catheterization, 74–76, **75;** after surgery, 96–98, 100, 106, 121–22, **122,** 136, 146–47, 151–52; for urinary retention, 74, 128, 146–47
Causes of incontinence, 2–3, 17–41
Cervix, 29; surgical removal of, 30
Cesarean delivery, 26
Childbirth: episiotomy for, 27, 167; incontinence after, 17, 23–26, **25,** 51
Clean intermittent self-catheterization, 74–76, **75,** 143; after augmentation cystoplasty, 120; after collagen injection, 91; difficulty with, 128–29, 146–47; after incontinence surgery, 98, 123, 146–47, 149, 151–52
Collagen (Contigen) injections, 88–91, **90,** 93, 94, 128, 134, 139
Colorectal surgeon, 43
Complications of treatment, 131, 136, 145–61; erosion or infection from synthetic materials, 156–58; fistula development, 153–55, **154;** kidney obstruction, 159–60; new pain, 160–61; persistent or new urgency or urge incontinence, 158–59; persistent or recurrent incontinence, 150–52; urinary retention, 145–50; urinary tract infection, 152–53
Connective tissues, 19, 39–40, 166

Consent for surgery, 135
Constipation, 19, 40
Consulting a doctor, 42–55, 162–64; assessing your situation and selecting the next step, 54; becoming a partner in your care, 45–46, 125–26, 163; bringing medical records, 51; finding the right doctor, 42–45, 162–63; first appointment with specialist, 47–48; having someone accompany you, 46–47; identifying best approach for you, 46–47 (*see also* Selecting treatment); physical examination, 48, 52–54; preparing for appointment, 46, 48–51; questions to ask, 51–52; taking medical history, 47–48; taking notes, 46
Contigen, 88
Coping with incontinence, 2, 42
Coughing, 17–19, 40, 53, 92, 93, 126
Cystocele, 27, **28,** 166
Cystometrogram, 59, 166
Cystoscopy, 56, 63–65, **64,** 166
Cystourethrocele, 27, 166

Darifenacin, 86
Decisions about treatment, 45–47, 125–27, 164
Dementia, 40, 92, 138
Desmopressin, 87–88
Detrol (tolterodine), 85–86, 159
Diabetes mellitus, 32–33, 40
Diapers, **69,** 69–71, 138–40
Dipstick test, 57
Ditropan (oxybutynin), 84–86, 159
Diuretic medications, 33, 88
Doctor visits. *See* Consulting a doctor
Duloxetine, 86
Dura-Sphere, 92

Elderly women, 138–40

Embarrassment, 3, 4, 44, 48, 49, 53, 82, 164

Embolus, 166–67

Endoscope, 167

Enterocele, **28,** 29, 167

Enterostomal therapist, 121

Enuresis, 20, 38–39, 87, 167

Epidural anesthesia, 100, 167

Episiotomy, 27, 167

Epispadias, 16

Erosion or infection from synthetic materials, 156–58

Estrogen, 10, 19, 31–32, 39

Estrogen replacement therapy, 32

Expectations of treatment, 5–6, 127–29, 163

External collecting bag, 116–18, **117**

Fecal incontinence, 137–38

Fibroids, uterine, 22–23, 30, 167

Finding the right doctor, 42–45, 162–63

Fistulas, 16, 31, 37–38, 153–55, **154,** 168

Flavoxate (Urispas), 85–86

Fluid intake, 49, 54, 83

Foley catheter, 31, 73–74, 98, 106, 121, 128–29, 146, 147, 168

Foreign object in urinary tract, 152–53

Frequent urination, 21–22, 32, 38, 54

Gastroenterologist, 43

General anesthesia, 63–64, 96, 105, 165

Glossary, 165–72

Goals of treatment, 5–6, 127–29, 163

Gynecologist, 43, 47, 56, 63, 96

Homografts, 107, 110, 168

Hyoscyamine (Levsin), 86

Hypnotherapy, 82–83

Hysterectomy, 29, 30–31, 37, 168; at time of incontinence surgery, 141; vesicovaginal fistula after, 153–55, **154**

Ileal conduit, 116

Imaging, 37, 56, 62, 65–66

Imipramine (Tofranil), 87

Implanted devices, 113–15; artificial urinary sphincter, 113–14, **114**; InterStim therapy, 114–15

Incontinence. *See* Fecal incontinence; Urinary incontinence

Infection: bladder, 20, 22, 27; from synthetic materials, 156–58; urinary tract, 20, 27, 40, 43, 121, 142, 152–53

Informed consent, 135

Injectable bulking agents, 63, 88–93, **90**

InterStim device, 114–15, 138

Interstitial cystitis, 59, 120, 168

Kegel exercises, 11–12, 76–77, 126–27

Kelly plication, 104–5, 146

Kidneys, 7–9, **8**; aging and function of, 39; obstructed, 159–60

Laparoscopic surgery, 111–13, 168

Laughing, 17, 18, 126

Leak point pressure test, 61–62

Learning about incontinence, 4–5, 45, 163

Levator muscles, 11, **11**

Levsin (hyoscyamine), 86

Lifestyle modifications, 83

Ligaments, **8,** 9, **14**; hysterectomy and, 31

Local anesthesia, 63, 106, 115, 165

Magnetic resonance imaging (MRI), 37, 56, 65, 66, 168

Magnetic stimulation, 81–82

Marshall-Marchetti-Krantz urethral suspension, 96, **101**, 101–2, 148

Medical history, 47–48

Medical tests, 48, 56–67

Medications: to alter urine odor, 71; antibiotics, 43, 58, 62, 65, 121, 142; diuretics, 33, 88; incontinence caused by, 54; for urinary retention, 146

Medications for incontinence, 83–88, 94, 134; combined stress incontinence and bladder overactivity, 87; how they work, 83; to reduce urine production, 87–88; side effects of, 84; stress incontinence, 86; tolerance to, 84; urge incontinence, 84–86, 159

Medline Plus, 173

Menopause, 10, 17, 31–32

Mixed incontinence, 16, 20, 32, 158–59, 168

Multiple sclerosis, 20, 33, 38, 143

Muscle contraction biofeedback, 81

Muscles: brain control of, 12–13, 15; changes with aging, 39; estrogen and strength of, 32; pelvic-floor, 7, **11**, 11–13; smooth (involuntary), 9–10, 12–13, 170; striated (voluntary), 9–13, 170

National Association for Continence, 45, 174

National Association for Home Care and Hospice, 173

National Institutes of Health, 174

National Kidney and Urologic Diseases Information Clearinghouse, 174

National Women's Health Information Center, 174

National Women's Health Resource Center, 174

Needle bladder neck suspension, 96, 103–4

Nerves: aging and function of, 40; during childbirth, 24; control of bladder function, 12–13, **13,** 15; damage due to bladder overstretching, 98; damage during hysterectomy, 30–31; sacral agenesis and, 36

Neurological disorders, 20, 33–39; due to pelvic operations and injuries, 37–38; enuresis and, 38–39; multiple sclerosis, 20, 33, 38, 143; Parkinson disease, 20, 38; spina bifida, 36–37, 123; spinal cord injury, 35–36; spinal cord tumors, 33; spinal stenosis, 33, 37; stroke, brain injury, and brain tumor, 33–35, **34**

Neurological examination, 52, 143

Neurologist, 43

Nocturia, 20, 32, 39, 49, 169

Nonsurgical treatments, 68–93; absorbent pads, 68–71, **69**; biofeedback techniques, 77–82, **79, 81**; catheters and clean intermittent self-catheterization, 73–76, **75**; hypnosis, 82–83; injectable bulking agents, 63, 88–93, **90**; lifestyle modifications, 83; medications, 83–88; pelvic-floor muscle exercises, 11–12, 26, 76–77; plugs and pessaries, 71–73, **72**

Nursing home admission, 1, 138

Ornade (phenylpropanolamine), 86

Ovaries: at menopause, 31; surgical removal of, 32

Overactive bladder, 21–22, 41, 151, 169; medications for, 87

Overflow incontinence, 16, 21, 33, 36, 37, 40, 41, 128, 169; catheterization for, 74; after surgery, 151

Overweight, 3, 128

Oxybutynin (Ditropan), 84–86, 159

Oxytrol, 85

Pad-weighing test, 56, 58

Pain after surgery, 160–61

Parkinson disease, 20, 38

Pelvic examination, 53

Pelvic-floor muscles, 7, **11,** 11–13, 169; examination of, 53; exercises for, 11–12, 26, 76–77, 126–27, 139

Pelvic nerve, 12, **13,** 169

Pelvic operations and injuries, 37–38

Pelvic organ prolapse, 11, 17, 26–29, **28, 30,** 169; pessaries for, **72,** 72–73; surgical correction of, 141

Pereyra suspension, 104

Perineum, 24, 169; examination of, 53; skin care, 70–71, 139, 140

Persistent incontinence after surgery, 150–52

Pessary, **72,** 72–73, 94, 169

Phenylpropanolamine (Ornade), 86

Physical examination, 48, 52–54

Physical therapist, 44

Pregnancy, 66; incontinence and, 18, 22–26, **23, 25,** 51; incontinence treatments and, 140

Pressure biofeedback, 80–81, **81**

Pressure-flow test, 59

Primary-care physician, 42–44

Pro-Banthine (propantheline), 86

Progesterone, 24, 31

Prolapse, 11, 17, 26–29, **28, 30,** 169; pessaries for, **72,** 72–73; surgical correction of, 141

Propantheline (Pro-Banthine), 86

Pseudoephedrine (Sudafed), 86

Pubic bone, **8,** 11, **14, 25,** 169

Pudendal nerve, 12, **13,** 169

Radiation therapy, 41, 108, 142

Raz suspension, 104

Rectocele, 27–29, **28,** 169

Rectum, 7, **8,** 11, **28,** 170; examination of, 53–54

Recurrent incontinence after surgery, 150–52

Research trial participation, 143–44

Residual volume test, 148

Resources, 4, 45–46, 173–75

Retention. *See* Urinary retention

Sacral agenesis, 36–37

Saddle anesthesia, 36

Selecting treatment, 46–47, 125–44, 163–64; with correction of pelvic organ prolapse, 141; for elderly woman, 138–40; future pregnancy and, 140; goals and expectations, 5–6, 127–29, 163; issues to consider in, 129–34; limitations from other conditions and, 141–43; opting for surgery, 135–38; research trial participation and, 143–44; with simultaneous hysterectomy, 141

Significance of incontinence, 1–2

Silicone particle injections, 92

Simon Foundation for Continence, 175

Skin care, perineal, 70–71, 139, 140

Sling operations, 95, **95,** 104–11, 123, 134, 170; bladder management after, 106–7; erosion or infection from synthetic materials used in,

Sling operations (continued)
156–58; Kelly plication, 104–5;
laparoscopic, 112; procedure for,
105–6, **106**; sources of tissues for,
107–10; tension-free vaginal tape,
110–11, 156
Smooth muscle, 9–10, 12–13, 170
Sneezing, 17, 18, 126
Society of Gynecologic Surgeons,
175
Solifenacin, 86
Specialist physicians, 43; first
appointment with, 47–48
Speculum, 53, 170
Spina bifida, 36–37, 123
Spinal anesthesia, 96, 100, 105
Spinal cord injury, 35–36
Spinal stenosis, 33, 37
Stamey suspension, 104
Stoma, 116–18, **117,** 121, 170
Stones, urinary, 153
Straight catheter, 73, 98, 121, **122,**
170
Stress incontinence, 16, 17–19,
**18,** 170; medications for, 86–87;
urinary retention after surgery
for, 145–50
Striated muscles, 9–13, 170
Stroke, 20, 34–35
Sudafed (pseudoephedrine), 86
Support groups, 4, 164
Suprapubic catheter, 74, 106, 146,
147, 170
Surgical treatments, 94–124; artificial
urinary sphincter, 113–14, **114;**
bladder management after, 97–98,
106–7, 121–23, **122;** categories of,
94–96; erosion or infection from
synthetic materials for, 156–58;
fistula development after, 153–55,

**154;** hysterectomy and, 141; informed consent for, 135; InterStim
therapy, 114–15, 138; laparoscopic,
111–13; new pain after, 160; obstructed kidney after, 159–60;
opting for, 135–38; persistent or
recurrent incontinence after,
150–52; questions to ask about,
135–37; sling operations, 95, **95,**
104–11, 170; suspension operations, 94, **95,** 96–104; urgency or
urge incontinence after, 158–59;
urinary diversion and reconstruction, 115–21, **117, 119;** urinary
retention after, 145–50; urinary
tract infection after, 152–53
Suspension operations, 94, **95,** 96–104,
170; bladder management after,
97–99, 145–50; Burch vaginal suspension, 96, 102–3, **103;** laparoscopic, 112; Marshall-Marchetti-
Krantz urethral suspension, 96,
**101,** 101–2; needle bladder neck
suspension, 96, 103–4; preparation
for, 99–100; procedure for, 96–97,
100
Sutures, 96–97, 101, 102, 170
Synthetic materials: erosion or infection from, 156–58; for slings,
109–10; tension-free vaginal tape,
110–11, 156

Tampons, 71–72, 73
Teflon injections, 91–92
Tension-free vaginal tape, 110–11,
156
Thrombus, 171
Tofranil (imipramine), 87
Toilet training, 15
Tolterodine (Detrol), 85–86, 159

Treatment: complications of, 131, 145–61; goals and expectations for, 5–6, 127–29, 163; locations for, 133; making decisions about, 45–47, 125–27, 164; nonsurgical, 68–93; options for, 4, 125, 130, 163–64; risks and benefits of, 131–32; selection of, 46–47, 125–44; success of, 132–33; surgical, 94–124, 135–38

Trospium, 86

Types of incontinence, 16–21

Ultrasound, 56, 62, 65, 66

Ureters, 7, **8,** 9, 171; damage during surgery, 159

Urethra, 7, **8,** 9, 10, 13–14, **14, 28;** during childbirth, 24, **25;** diverticulum of, 16, 171; in epispadias, 16; vaginal mobility and weakness of, 29, **30**

Urethral cap, patch, or plug, 71

Urethral pressure profile, 62

Urethral sphincter, 7, **8,** 10, **11,** 12, 14, 171; aging and function of, 40; artificial, 113–14, **114;** spinal cord injury and, 35–36; weakness of, 17

Urethrocele, 27, **28,** 171

Urethrolysis, 150

Urethroscopy, 171

Urethrovaginal fistula, **154,** 155

Urge incontinence, 16, 19–20, 38, 171; medications for, 84–86, 159; after surgery, 122, 134, 136, 158–59

Urgency, 19–20, 21–22, 27, 32, 35, 38, 138, 158–59

Urinalysis, 48, 56–58, 171

Urinary diversion and reconstruction, 115–21; augmentation cystoplasty, 118–20, **119;** Bricker diversion, 116–18, **117**

Urinary flow rate test, 147–48

Urinary incontinence: causes of, 2–3, 17–41; consulting a doctor about, 42–55, 162–64; definition of, 1; learning about, 4–5, 45, 163; mixed, 16, 20, 32, 158–59, 168; overflow, 16, 21, 33, 36, 37, 40, 41, 169; significance of, 1–2; stress, 16, 17–19, **18,** 86–87, 170; taking control of, 162–64; treatment of (*See* Treatment); types of, 16–21; urge, 16, 19–20, 38, 84–86, 158–59, 171; what to do about, 3–6

Urinary retention, 37, 171; catheterization for, 74, 128, 146–47; after collagen injection, 90–91, 128; after surgery, 145–50

Urinary tract, 7–15, **8;** brain and, 33–34, **34;** changes with aging, 39–40; examination of, 52–54; foreign object in, 152–53; stones in, 153

Urinary tract infection, 20, 27, 40, 43, 121, 142; after surgery, 152–53

Urination, 14; altering habits of, 54; in diabetes, 32–33; after surgery, 97–98, 106–7, 121–22, 145–50

Urine, 7–9; medications to alter odor of, 71; medications to reduce production of, 87–88

Urispas (flavoxate), 85–86

Urodynamic test, 56, 58–62, **60,** 171–72

Urogynecologist, 43

Urologist, 43, 44, 47, 56, 63, 82, 96, 142

Uterus, **8,** 26, **28,** 172; fibroids in, 22–23, 30, 167; in pregnancy, 24; prolapse of, **28,** 29; surgical removal of, 29, 30–31, 168

Vagina, 7, **8,** 11, **14,** 26, **28,** 172; urethral weakness and mobility of, 29, **30**
Vaginal cones, 80, **81,** 139
Vaginal probe, 80–81

Vaginal vault prolapse, 29
Vesicovaginal fistula, 16, 153–55, **154**
Vulva, 53, 172

"Water pills," 33

Xenografts, 108, 109, 172
X-rays, 37, 56, 62, 65–66

## About the Authors

**Rene Genadry** has been at the Johns Hopkins Medical Institutions since 1971. He is currently an associate professor in the Department of Gynecology and Obstetrics and has a private practice in gynecology, urogynecology, and pelvic reconstructive surgery. He received an M.D. from the French Faculty of Medicine and completed his residency at the Johns Hopkins Hospital. For 25 years he has organized and directed the annual Houston Everett Memorial Course in Urogynecology, which teaches updated knowledge and techniques to thousands of practicing urologists and gynecologists on subjects of urinary and fecal incontinence, pelvic prolapse, and gynecological surgery. He has been a director of the Division of Gynecology at Johns Hopkins and a member of the board of directors of the American Urogynecological Society. Most recently, he organized an international consensus conference on the prevention and treatment of obstetrical fistula in the developing world in conjunction with the Bill and Melinda Gates Institute at the Johns Hopkins Bloomberg School of Public Health.

**Jacek L. Mostwin** has been at Johns Hopkins since 1978. He is currently professor of urology in the Brady Urological Institute, where he is also director of the Division of Reconstructive and Neurological Urology. He received a B.S. from Tufts College, an M.D. from the University of Maryland, and a D.Phil. from the University of Oxford. He has served as chairman of the Pathophysiology Subcommittee of the World Health Organization's International Consultation in Incontinence and as a member of the American Urological Association's Committee on Guidelines for Stress Incontinence Surgery, and he is currently a member of the editorial board of the journal *Neurourology and Urodynamics*. In addition to his clinical experience, he has made contributions to the scientific study of the smooth muscle of the urinary bladder and is a director of the School of Medicine's course entitled "Patient, Physician and Society." He has collaborated with Dr. Genadry in the Houston Everett Course for the past 20 years.